HIS MOTHER
CALLED HIM

YESHUA

THE WORLD
CALLS HIM

JESUS

Hearts

What Are They? How They Work?

Betty Ames

Bloomington, IN 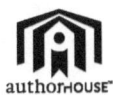 authorHOUSE™ Milton Keynes, UK

AuthorHouse™
1663 Liberty Drive, Suite 200
Bloomington, IN 47403
www.authorhouse.com
Phone: 1-800-839-8640

First published by AuthorHouse 9/14/2007

ISBN#: 1-4259-3870-1

Printed in the United States of America
Bloomington, Indiana

This book is printed on acid-free paper.

'HEARTS' has been written to:

1. Give GOD Glory for the great and mighty things HE has carried me through and taught me by the Fire of HIS HOLY SPIRIT.

2. Thank HIM for the wonderful and precious gifts HE has given me in each of my six children, Ted, Edward, Ronni, Jimmy and Chris, & Jerome their spouse and each of my fifteen { grand-children} Joshua, Wesley, Joseph, Michael, David, Amanda, Tracie, Elizabeth, Daniel, Taylor, Tara, Jonathan, Rachel, Charity & Teddie who were each born perfectly in HIS IMAGE, and for any future blessings HE feels I deserve.

3. Thank HIM for my wonderful Parents who did their very best to raise me in a Christian home and who loved me inspite of myself and my rebellion. For my two brothers and my sister and their children.

4. Thank HIM for a husband who, inspite of his condition, supports all that I do and loves me even when I am wrong.

5. Baruch Ha Shem {Bless the NAME}, my Messianic Congregation where I have found fulfillment in the teachings of my Rabbi Marty Waldman & the 'Leaders' as well as the agape'love' I have found there from them and all my wonderful sisters and brothers

DISCLAIMER

This study, "STATE OF OUR HEART" is not meant to arouse one to ever attempt to walk by faith with out having a vast knowledge of GOD'S WORD, which none of us ever really completely have while we sojourn here. But GOD'S blessings to us include HIS PRECIOUS HOLY SPIRIT who will teach us precept upon precept, brick upon brick to become seasoned in HIS WORD, seeking HIS FACE and knowing beyond any doubt that HE alone is able to deliver.

Great caution is pleaded and heeded for anyone reading State of our Heart. AND warning is hereby given, NOT to withdraw from using medical prescriptions given by the 'Doctor' that are helpful to the body, for GOD has also placed many Doctors in positions of ministry and when they are GODLY Doctors the patient will be blessed and comforted.

'STATE OF OUR HEART' was given over a period of years and written to explain major areas of faith, and to encourage one to begin to search the SCRIPTURE for answers.

Only the SCRIPTURES are alive with compassion and healing as well as justice. These items are issued from the same fountain and can not be separated.

Only when The SCRIPTURES are absorbed, digested, inhaled, thought and lived will they diagnose, treat and cure problems. And only those, whose HEART is open and comes alive under "HIS WORD", will realize the power and preparation initiated by the procedures of the Contents.

There are no short cuts or other directions to reach GOD, apart from YESHUA {JESUS}. It was only YESHUA, who made the offering of death for our sin and became our Perfect SACRIFICE.

For all who are unwilling to read, study, absorb, drink of the Living Water {SCRIPTURE}, and eat of the Bread of Life {SCRIPTURE} there is no life.

The Author of 'HEARTS' assumes no responsibility for adverse effects or consequences for anyone who reads 'STATE OF OUR HEART' and hereby issues this WARNING: To stop taking your physicians advice is unthinkable with out full knowledge of GOD, and only you are capable of making such a decision. We are called to make every moment count in the dynamic consciousness and delight of living vigorously by abiding in and of 'The SCRIPTURE'

Contents

HEART STRUCTURE

The HEART is delicate and durable and embroidered with vessels, it circulates the blood and sustains the body's 60,000-mile cardiovascular system. It is an eleven-ounce pump that issues power and creates life for mankind.

This VITAL ORGAN lies inside the chest beneath the breastbone, and is a simple yet astonishing organ that is merely a muscle but no less a fountain of life. In form it is a hollow, pear-shaped bag, separated from top to bottom by a wall of tissue. Each side possesses a small, upper chamber called the atrium and a larger, lower chamber known as the ventricle. Connecting the two chambers is a valve that forces blood to flow in only one direction, from the atria to the ventricles and from the ventricles out of the HEART. In a healthy HEART no blood passes directly between the left and right halves. As simple as it seems, the HEART is the core of life.

This SEAT OF PASSION is a life-giving pump but for mankind it is a simple machine with a sacred mission. Its labor is brute, its fabric coarse, yet it connects and sustains the body's work.

Cardiac rhythm allows the brain [computer] to think, the lungs to breathe and the muscles to move.

The HEART is the pivot of life and provides the truth about mans inter-most desires to GOD, it is GOD'S link to mortal man. What is concealed in the HEART will be the ruler of our time on earth and establish our eternal destination. A seventeen century physician named <u>William Harvey</u> proclaimed with certainty that the HEART is 'the sovereign' of the body.

Long ago the discovery of circulation traced the blood's surging force to the pump action of the HEART. But little was known about the force itself until Stephen Hales, an eighteenth-century English pastor who made the first accurate measurements of blood pressure. While Hales attended Cambridge University he developed a passion for science and pursued anatomical wisdom as he deftly moved between the worlds of dutiful minister and daring scientist. The transition was easy; he saw one job as an extension of the other. Hales felt the study of the works of GOD revealed the Signatures of HIS wisdom and power in everything.

The HEART kindles and fulfills life's flame and consequently motivates man's wonderment. In the beginning of life at the fourth week of pregnancy, a concentration of cells inside the developing embryo suddenly acquires purpose. Inexplicably, the cells begin to pulse, sparking a rhythm that will carry throughout life.

Greek philosopher <u>Aristotle</u> thought the HEART to be the first organ to live and the last to die, an organ from which 'the motions of the body commence.'

To <u>Leonardo da Vinci</u>, lifelong student of anatomy, the HEART spoke, if not volumes, then close to it: "With what words will you describe this HEART, so as not to fill a book...?" He reasoned that the HEART'S pumping action, the rush of blood through valves and vessels, generated body heat in the same manner that churning warmed freshly made butter. Blood in the HEART must be warm, he said, in order for the 'vivifying' process, the bringing of life to the tissues to work. "The tears come from the HEART, not the brain." He wrote. He was a observer in the field of anatomy.

HEART surgery preceding 1930 was considered relative to medical heresy. Of all the vital parts of the body the HEART is the simplest but it was the last the scalpel dared to touch. Perhaps what kept the HEART so long undisturbed was man's sense that to cut this organ meant to cut too close to the quick of life.

To the ancients, the HEART contained the spiritual essence of man while the Egyptians weighed the HEART of the dead to measure truth and the Greeks saw the HEART as a forge, burning impurities from the blood. Centuries later, when the wheel of science began to turn faster and man learned to move water, he recast this mysterious organ in a new found image. The HEART became known as a pump.

Modern diagnostic tools have given the HEART a thousand faces and its anatomy has become artistry through the magic of X-rays, computers and video equipment.

In 1953 a Texas surgeon Michael DeBakey designed a machine that could manufacture a seamless, knit Dacron tube that would provide the means to insert artificial arteries where needed. He was a pioneer who took bold steps that opened a forbidden territory to build the ultimate of gadgets, an artificial HEART. DeBakey demanded perfection and set an example few can match; he often worked 24 hour days, a compassionate man who deeply mourns the loss of a patient. Even so there are no doctors who have any control over human life but GOD for the soul is eternal, not the fleshly body.

Man's medical inventiveness has reached inside the chest and touched the human HEART. For minutes, hours or, in some cases years physicians can make metal, plastic and electricity do the work of muscle, fiber and nerve. Devices like the auxiliary ventricle can temporarily ease the HEART'S workload and give the HEART the chance to heal itself. GOD is the giver of health and life and when we do not know HIM we walk as the dead wasting space and air.

Today, men know the HEART as a technical masterpiece and timeless metaphor. From it springs life bound to the virtues of honor, love and courage. The HEART ties body to spirit, the mystical past to the practical present and is an observation of focus for GOD to examine our convictions.

In this time giants of HEART research who are not content to explore with their hands, eyes and ears have turned to instruments such as the X-ray and the electrocardiograph and have discovered various ways to approach the HEART with human diagnosed rationale but the root problem of all dis-ease of humankind is transgression, better known as sin in simplistic terminology. The sin of mankind has become satan's weapon to exercise offense to contrast a Supreme GOD. In other words, it is satan's only method to subject GOD to sorrow and lamentation through the abuse of HIS Created Image, MAN.

"A merry HEART maketh a cheerful countenance", is counsel from the Book of Proverbs, "but by sorrow of the HEART the spirit is broken." In language, this VITAL ORGAN not only breaks but it sings, turns as hard as stone, becomes heavy or light, cold or warm. Character may be drawn from the pure of HEART, the kindhearted, the hale and hearty of the bleeding HEART. To speak from the bottom of the HEART epitomizes sincerity and whatever the HEART is full of will reflect in the flesh. If the HEART is full of evil it will harden and the demeanor will reflect evil and darkness but if the HEART is pure it will reflect happiness, trust and joy.

HEARTS were created and intended by the SUPREME CREATOR to perform and fulfill HIS WILL and is the dwelling place for HIM to inhabit and influence our passage, intention and existence. Therefore, each HEART can only comprehend fulfillment when there is a submissive dependence on the Almighty GOD. The actuality is that many of us are blinded to HIS wondrous genuineness and light as we flounder in ignorance, aggrieved and distressed serving HIS enemy satan, the attacker of our soul.

Unfortunately, in these times, many have experienced worthless, empty traditions and counterfeit acts of righteousness by peers, counselors or clergyman and women an even priest.

Accomplishments that seem real but have in fact caused us to miss the mark, clouded our rationalization and have left us with a superficial fraudulent GOSPEL. Thus we have misunderstood the uncomplicated and simple meaning of HIS WORD that grants angelic protection. HIS MIGHTY ANGELS will establish an invisible shield on every side of those who serve HIM with their whole HEART.

PSALMS 34:7 HERE WAS A LOWLY MAN WHO CALLED, AND THE LORD LISTENED, AND DELIVERED HIM FROM ALL HIS TROUBLES. :8 THE ANGEL OF THE LORD CAMPS AROUND THOSE WHO FEAR HIM AND RESCUES THEM.

PSALMS 35:4 LET THOSE WHO SEEK MY LIFE BE FRUSTRATED AND PUT TO SHAME; LET THOSE WHO PLAN TO HARM ME FALL BACK IN DISGRACE. :5 LET THEM BE AS CHAFF IN THE WIND, THE LORD'S ANGEL DRIVING THEM ON. JEWISH TANAKH

PSALMS 40:9 TO DO WHAT PLEASES YOU, MY GOD, IS MY DESIRE. YOUR TEACHING IS IN MY INMOST PARTS. [HEART] JEWISH TANAKH

Today America has turned HER HEART from GOD as She promenades in the arrogant haughtiness of HER history when GOD was Her Leader and She was a virtuous and ethical Nation that cared for Her Own. Our performance and apathy have caused America's magnificence to diminish as temples are built to glorify false god's made of stone or wood or SELF until now when America wallows in the ooze of foreign and corrupt Nations who have come in with their counterfeit and puny gods to destroy even the meaning of what America previously stood for.

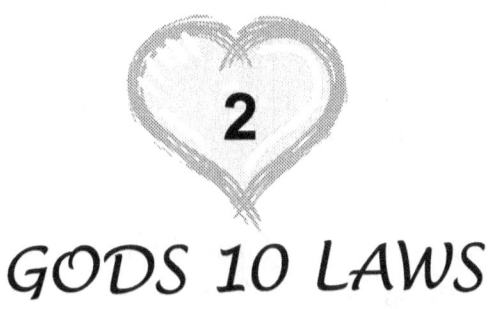

GODS 10 LAWS

As GOD gave MOSES the 10 GREAT COMMANDMENTS HIS FIRST ONE concerned other gods. Consequently, we find that the ONE and ONLY TRUE GOD is a jealous GOD and rightfully so as the CREATOR of all made in HIS IMAGE, HE, WHO has numbered even the hairs on our head and sees into each HEART. The same GOD WHO divides the bone and marrow can also separate the body from the soul. Is there another 'god' so majestic as HE that has done so much or is competent to deliver us from satan the enemy?

The FIRST GREAT COMMANDMENT says:

EXODUS 20:3-17 I THE LORD AM YOUR GOD WHO BROUGHT YOU OUT OF EGYPT, THE HOUSE OF BONDAGE :3 YOU SHALL <u>HAVE NO OTHER gods</u> BEFORE ME :4 YOU <u>SHALL NOT</u> MAKE FOR YOURSELF A SCULPTURED IMAGE, OR ANY LIKENESS OF WHAT IS IN THE HEAVENS ABOVE, OR ON THE EARTH BELOW, OR IN THE WATERS UNDER THE EARTH: YOU SHALL <u>NOT BOW DOWN</u> TO

THEM OR SERVE THEM. FOR I THE LORD YOUR GOD AM AN IMPASSIONED GOD, VISITING THE GUILT OF THE PARENTS UPON THE CHILDREN, UPON THE THIRD AND UPON THE FOURTH GENERATIONS OF THOSE WHO REJECT ME :6 BUT SHOWING KINDNESS TO THE THOUSANDTH GENERATION OF THOSE WHO LOVE ME AND KEEP MY COMMANDMENTS. :7 YOU SHALL NOT SWEAR FALSELY BY THE NAME OF THE LORD YOUR GOD; FOR THE LORD WILL NOT CLEAR ONE WHO SWEARS FALSELY BY HIS NAMES. JEWISH TANAKH   DEUT. 5:7-21 YE SHALL HAVE NO OTHER gods BEFORE ME   JEWISH TANAKH

Egypt in today's term is a form of bondage also of the world and when GOD brings us out of darkness it is likened to coming out of Egypt. In effect we all pass from the bondage of death to life through GOD'S benevolent mercy to become free.

In the TANAKH {Old Testament, Covenant} GOD came down to visit with Moses at Mount Sinai and wrote HIS DIVINE LAW, the 10 COMMANDMENTS on Tablets of Stone with the DIVINE FIRE of HIS HOLY SPIRIT.

In the New Testament {Covenant} GOD sent the DIVINE ROCK in YESHUA, the INCARNATE WORD to live and walk among us in human form, not above us. YESHUA came willingly, knowing HE would be the ultimate sacrifice for our sin but HE would also be the authentic Cloak [covering] for everyone to enter into Heaven as HIS BLOOD covered our transgression so that we can be counted as worthy to go before The Heavenly FATHER. HE proved HIS sympathetic and miraculous love for us when HE carried our transgressions and iniquities into hell on HIS back and left them so that through HIM we would have victory over our sin by seeking HIS WILL for our lives. Those who confess and receive GOD become HIS Child by adoption and instantly become worthy to have the same DIVINE LAW that heals and brings new life written upon the tablets of the HEART just as GOD did at the festival of Shavu'ot {feast of weeks} in:

ACTS 2:2 SUDDENLY THERE CAME A SOUND FROM THE SKY LIKE THE ROAR OF A VIOLENT WIND, AND IT FILLED THE WHOLE HOUSE WHERE THEY WERE SITTING. :3 THEN THEY SAW WHAT LOOKED LIKE TONGUES OF FIRE, WHICH SEPARATED AND CAME TO REST ON EACH ONE OF THEM :4 THEY WERE ALL FILLED WITH THE RUACH HAKODESH {HOLY SPIRIT} AND BEGAN TO TALK IN DIFFERENT LANGUAGES, AS THE SPIRIT ENABLED THEM TO SPEAK. JEWISH NEW TESTAMENT

In Acts 2:4 the message entered the HEART, being written there with the same DIVINE FIRE from above that forged the TEN COMMANDMENTS onto the ROCK at Mount Sinai and will be ever lasting.

We should never take for granted that precious LAW given by GOD to Moses on the Mountain for it was meant to be the moral code for all of humanity. This moral code is the revelation of GOD'S LAW, the social code is the regulation of that Law and the spiritual code is the realization of that Law in and through YESHUA as HE said in:

MATTHEW 5:17 DON'T THINK THAT I HAVE COME TO ABOLISH THE TORAH {LAW} OR THE PROPHETS. I HAVE COME NOT TO ABOLISH BUT TO COMPLETE. JEWISH NEW TESTAMENT

As American's stand in awe and wonderment of what has happened we are being raped and plundered due to our own stubbornness and blindness. Our pride and selfishness have flourished as America stands as a Nation that has forgotten the ONE and ONLY TRUE GOD of all gods, LORD of all lords and KING of all kings. The essential quality of America has been lost and Her HEART has turned to stone. Today HEART attacks on

America are a constant rhythm in the form of crime, hunger, weather and catastrophes sent from GOD'S treasures that now strike the very foundation of what was once a great and mighty Nation where GOD'S WAYS and GOD'S DAY was honored and important. Where once the LORD'S day was reverenced and cherished, today it is scorned and abused. America walks in deceit and rebellion against GOD and is now in bondage, even so in HIS Great wondrous mercy there is still hope.

If the people of America who claim to be 'Christian' or just those who attend a BIBLE believing congregation would humble themselves, repent, pray and seek GOD'S FACE, HE would hear and HE would repent [seek compassion] and save our Nation as described in:

2 CHRONICLES 7:14 WHEN MY PEOPLE, WHO BEAR MY NAME, HUMBLE THEMSELVES, PRAY AND SEEK MY FAVOR AND TURN FROM THEIR EVIL WAYS, I WILL HEAR IN MY HEAVENLY ABODE AND FORGIVE THEIR SIN AND HEAL THEIR LAND. JEWISH TANAKH

2 CORINTHIANS 3:16 BUT, SAYS THE TORAH [OLD TESTAMENT], WHENEVER SOMEONE TURNS TO ADONAI [THE LORD, JEHOVAH] THE VEIL IS TAKEN AWAY. :17 NOW, AND WHERE THE SPIRIT OF ADONAI [THE LORD] IS, THERE IS FREEDOM. :18 SO ALL OF US, WITH FACES UNVEILED, SEE AS IN A MIRROR THE GLORY OF THE LORD; AND WE ARE BEING CHANGED INTO HIS VERY IMAGE, FROM ONE DEGREE OF GLORY TO THE NEXT, BY ADONAI THE SPIRIT. JEWISH NEW TESTAMENT

Why are HEART ATTACKS AND STROKES such a common occurrence in today's society? If our HEART is in GOD'S HAND and HE is in complete control and we are HIS CREATION, HIS Children, then as any good Father, should HE not expect HIS Children to obey HIM? Instead far to many sow seeds of rebellion and sin that can only reap the harvest of pain and suffering with in the HEART and life.

GOD has given to each of us free choice, a will to do as we please. Our 'selection' is the navigator of our time we spend here on earth. With in this frame of time we are given options or choices of what GOD or gods we elect to serve, our decision will be the forecaster of our victory or defeat here on earth as well determine where we will spend eternity.

Our Health is maintained by our decisions and actions which stem from the HEART. Should we or should we not tend to these temples {bodies} GOD has granted us title too?

There are numerous explanations for disease and every last one stem from the chief[HEART] of our temple[body] to harvest what has been sown.

PROVERBS 18:6 THE WORDS OF A FOOL LEAD TO STRIFE; HIS SPEECH INVITES <u>BLOWS {STROKES}</u> JEWISH TANAKH

EZEKIEL 24:13 FOR YOUR VILE IMPURITY, BECAUSE I SOUGHT TO CLEANSE YOU OF <u>YOUR IMPURITY</u>, BUT YOU WOULD NOT BE CLEANSED {REBELLION} YOU SHALL NEVER BE CLEAN AGAIN UNTIL I HAVE <u>SATISFIED MY FURY UPON YOU</u>. :14 I THE LORD HAVE SPOKEN; IT SHALL COME TO PASS AND I WILL DO IT. I WILL NOT REFRAIN OR SPARE OR RELENT. YOU SHALL BE PUNISHED ACCORDING TO YOUR WAYS AND YOUR DEEDS, DECLARES THE LORD GOD. :15 THE WORD OF THE LORD CAME TO ME :16 O MORTAL, I AM ABOUT TO TAKE AWAY THE DELIGHT OF YOUR EYES FROM YOU THROUGH <u>PESTILENCE</u>; BUT YOU SHALL NOT LAMENT OR WEEP OR LET YOUR TEARS FLOW. :17 MOAN SOFTLY; OBSERVE NO MOURNING FOR THE DEAD. JEWISH TANAKH

EZK. 24:16 <u>I WILL TAKE THE DESIRES OF THINE HEART WITH A STROKE.</u> KING JAMES VERSION

HEBREWS 3:13 INSTEAD, KEEP EXHORTING EACH OTHER EVERY DAY, AS LONG AS IT IS CALLED TODAY, SO THAT NONE OF YOU WILL BECOME <u>HARDENED BY THE DECEIT OF SIN.</u> JEWISH NEW TESTAMENT HEBREWS 3:7 THEREFORE, AS THE RUACH HA KODESH {HOLY SPIRIT} SAYS, TODAY IF YOU HEAR GOD'S VOICE, :8 <u>DON'T HARDEN YOUR HEARTS,</u> AS YOU DID IN THE BITTER QUARREL ON THAT DAY IN THE WILDERNESS WHEN YOU PUT GOD TO THE TEST. JEWISH NEW TESTAMENT

When we mature in HIS WORD we see in SCRIPTURE how HE cautions <u>not to let our HEART become hard</u>. If we stand still and ponder that most HEART disease, attacks and the like are methodically induced by the rigid and hardened HEART perchance we will recognize that being in HIS WILL and PRESENCE is to anticipate the inheritance of health.

1 PETER 2:24 HE HIMSELF BORE OUR SIN IN HIS BODY ON THE STAKE, SO THAT WE MIGHT DIE TO SIN AND LIVE FOR RIGHTEOUSNESS, <u>BY HIS WOUNDS YOU WERE HEALED</u>. JEWISH NEW TESTAMENT our prayer daily

PSALMS 51:12 FASHION A PURE HEART FOR ME, O GOD, CREATE IN ME A STEADFAST SPIRIT :13 DON'T CAST ME OUT OF YOUR PRESENCE, OR TAKE YOUR HOLY SPIRIT AWAY FROM ME JEWISH TANAKH

As we examine GOD'S WORD we find that sin and rebellion are the root cause for defeat. We will also come to know and understand the preventive measures that will maintain and consecrate the HEART from becoming callous and sinking towards death. GOD is real, there is no dispute that HE was and is and will be forever more and HE assembled us in HIS IMAGE.

Once we begin to know HIM we will comprehend and appreciate to what end HE allows the dreadful pains and ill health befall us and those we love.

2 TIMOTHY 2:15 KJV SAYS 'STUDY TO SHOW OURSELVES APPROVED. JEWISH NEW TESTAMENT SAYS, 'DO ALL YOU CAN TO PRESENT YOURSELF TO GOD AS SOMEONE WORTHY OF HIS APPROVAL, AS A WORKER WITH NO NEED TO BE ASHAMED, BECAUSE HE DEALS STRAIGHT FORWARDLY WITH THE WORD OF THE TRUTH :16 KEEP AWAY FROM godless BABBLING, FOR THOSE WHO ENGAGE IN IT WILL ONLY BECOME MORE ungodly :17 THEIR TEACHING WILL EAT AWAY AT PEOPLE LIKE GANGRENE. :18 THEY HAVE MISSED THE MARK, AS FAR AS TRUTH IS CONCERNED. JEWISH NEW TESTAMENT

Each of us are born anathematize by the ancestral disobedience of Adam in the Garden of Eden and as a result we are guilty of sin because we are inbred with the curse of sin in our HEART. But GOD in HIS benevolence made provisions for children and does not hold them responsible until they come to the age of accountability to know the moral from immoral. Even as a child GOD forged right performance into our consciousness and gave us an awareness of morality that we must be accountable for, therefore we are expected to pursue good.

GOD gave each child a set of birth parents and called them mother and father and HE purposed them to direct, provide and be guardians up to an age of accountability, nevertheless these days the majority of parents do not recognize GOD, consequently America struggles with in to recapture Her previously celebrated status. At the same time satan recognizes Her moral condition and knows his time is short, he stalks about as a roaring lion seeking whom he may devour.

Many American's profess Salvation as if it were a part of their life yet it is lip service taken much to lightly and has become a blind spot to justify foolish fleshly desires. If the 'Christian' could not be brought down to miss Heaven, satan would have no reason to stalk about and cause even 'the elect' to fall.

1 PETER 5:8 STAY SOBER, STAY ALERT! YOUR ENEMY, THE ADVERSARY, STALKS ABOUT LIKE A ROARING LION LOOKING FOR SOMEONE TO DEVOUR   JEWISH NEW TESTAMENT

BY GOD'S DESIGN

The HEART is GOD'S MASTERPIECE, HE has full authority, our steps are ordained and ordered by HIM whether or not we are obedient to HIM or loyal to HIS archenemy, HE is in absolute dominance. HIS sovereignty can not and will not change, HE will render evil for evil and good for good.

When we repent and become faithful to acknowledge YESHUA'S life, death and resurrection, we unload our sin in repentance from a HEART that desires change, we will turn from evil to pursue GOD and in HIS compassion HE will forgive and forget our sin.

EZEKIEL 18:29b I WILL JUDGE EACH ONE OF YOU ACCORDING TO HIS WAYS, DECLARES THE LORD GOD. REPENT AND TURN BACK FROM YOUR TRANSGRESSIONS, LET THEM NOT BE A STUMBLING BLOCK OF GUILT FOR YOU. :31 CAST AWAY ALL THE TRANSGRESSIONS BY WHICH YOU HAVE OFFENDED, AND GET YOURSELVES A NEW HEART AND A NEW SPIRIT, THAT YOU MAY NOT

DIE. OH HOUSE OF ISRAEL. :32 FOR IT IS NOT MY DESIRE THAT ANYONE SHALL DIE, DECLARES THE LORD GOD, REPENT, THEREFORE AND LIVE. JEWISH TANAKH

SCRIPTURE displays a perpetual theme of GOD'S SALVATION and man's urgency to be sanctified. The purpose of life and the meaning of history is that GOD ransomed humanity from the wretchedness of sin and reinstated the conditions that enable individuals and nations to relate rightly with HIM. All Morality and happiness are inseparably linked with SALVATION.

JESUS' name was translated to English from the name YESHUA which means SALVATION in HEBREW. According to the TANAKH [OLD TESTAMENT] GOD created man to be in intimate, loving and obedient fellowship with HIM. Because of man's rebellion and choice to go his own way GOD made provision for man kind by commissioning HIS ONLY SON as the Perfect and Ultimate BLOOD sacrifice, a Cloak for our sin.

The word rebellion means sin and the punishment for sin is death, not only termination of life but everlasting separation from GOD. But GOD'S MERCY is impartial and HE wills to rescue all mankind from what we deserve. To consummate SALVATION for us GOD sent the MASHIACH [MESSIAH] translated to English the MASHIACH is CHRIST.

YESHUA [JESUS] was the SHEM [NAME] HE was known by in BIBLICAL TIMES. Christians later translated YESHUA to JESUS for the English speaking world and GOD acknowledges that translation for HIS ANOINTED SON and answers prayers in the NAME OF JESUS according to the attitude of our HEART. GOD is a discerner of the HEART and HE searches for confirmation of a pure HEART, one that hungers after HIS WILL and desires to serve HIM.

In HIS WORD many references can be found concerning the HEART that describe treasures of gold in threads of silver for our guidance, deliverance, abundant life and eternal SALVATION.

HEBREWS 4:12 THE WORD OF GOD IS ALIVE. IT IS AT WORK AND IS SHARPER THAN ANY DOUBLE EDGED SWORD. IT CUTS RIGHT THROUGH TO WHERE SOUL MEETS SPIRIT AND JOINTS MEET MARROW, AND IT IS QUICK TO JUDGE THE INNER REFLECTIONS AND ATTITUDES OF THE HEART :13 BEFORE GOD, NOTHING CREATED IS HIDDEN, BUT ALL THINGS ARE NAKED AND OPEN TO THE EYES OF HIM TO WHOM WE MUST RENDER ACCOUNT. JEWISH NEW TESTAMENT

FOLLOWING ARE <u>A FEW REFERENCES TO THE HEART FROM HIS WORD AND SHOULD BE TAKEN LITERALLY.</u>

*IF WE<u> REFUSE TO FORGIVE OTHERS, HE CAN'T FORGIVE US </u> MATTHEW 18:35

*DO NOT   LET OUR<u> HEART BE HARDENED</u> MARK 2:8; 10:5;16:14; MATTHEW 19:8; DEUT. 10:16; JER 4:4

*BE NOT TROUBLED BUT TRUST IN GOD   JOHN 14:1

*HE LEFT US WITH SHALOM {PEACE} NOT THE SHALOM OF THIS WORLD, DO NOT FEAR JOHN 14:27

*BLESSED ARE THE PURE IN HEART MATTHEW 5:8

*O LORD OF HOSTS, YOU WHO TEST THE RIGHTEOUS, WHO EXAMINE THE HEART AND THE MIND JERE. 20:12

*SAY TO THE ANXIOUS OF HEART, BE STRONG, FEAR NOT; BEHOLD YOUR GOD! ISAIAH 35:4

*IF YOU OBEY THE COMMANDMENTS THAT I ENJOIN UPON YOU THIS DAY, LOVING THE LORD YOUR GOD AND SERVING HIM WITH ALL YOUR HEART AND SOUL DEUTERONOMY 11:13

*I WILL REMOVE THE HEART OF STONE FROM THEIR BODIES AND GIVE THEM A HEART OF FLESH EZEKIEL 11:19

*BUT IF YOU HARBOR IN YOUR HEARTS BITTER JEALOUSY AND SELFISH AMBITION, DON'T BOAST AND ATTACK THE TRUTH WITH LIES JAMES 3:14

ALL REFERENCES ARE FROM JEWISH TANAKH OR JEWISH NEW TESTAMENT

Today strokes and HEART attacks are customary they are almost as common as a headache or the like. It seems the world has gone insane and souls are amassed in panic and fear. But why? Fear of what? Where GOD dwells there is:

PERFECT LOVE CASTETH OUT FEAR 1 JOHN 4:18

FEAR OF THE LORD IS THE BEGINNING OF KNOWLEDGE; BUT FOOLS DESPISE WISDOM AND DISCIPLINE. PROVERBS 1:7

Let us take into account creation, The CREATOR, WHO formed each to be different. He made us after HIS OWN IMAGE. HIS WHOLENESS and WILL are absolutely a part of HIS IMAGE and since HE is love, truth, justice, virtuous and in complete control, if we are in HIS Image, how could we be different?

ROMANS 1:19 BECAUSE WHAT IS KNOWN ABOUT GOD IS PLAIN TO THEM, SINCE GOD HAS MADE IT PLAIN TO THEM :20 FOR EVER SINCE THE CREATION OF THE

UNIVERSE HIS INVISIBLE QUALITIES, BOTH HIS ETERNAL POWER AND HIS DIVINE NATURE, HAVE BEEN CLEARLY SEEN, BECAUSE THEY CAN BE UNDERSTOOD FROM WHAT HE HAS MADE. THEREFORE THEY HAVE NO EXCUSE. JEWISH NEW TESTAMENT

The reality is, HE created each of us in a particular design in HIS IMAGE so in the event that we oppose HIS attributes that were naturally placed into our HEART, the HEART is powerless to confront or interpret them and immediately begins a resistance, a procedure of obstruction that eventually dulls our spiritual perception and turns to stone.

While resistance to evil is the HEART'S concept of protection, it is actually a satanic corruption of death for as the HEART with draws to resist the enemy it deliberately envelopes a defense to depravity and chances to become sightless by the rock of protection, hardened in hypocrisy so that the very life that is in the Blood can no longer flow freely. The stone of horror has crusted and overlaid an impenetrable film encasing this vital organ until there is no method of repair with out surgery or repentance for a new HEART.

1 SAMUEL 10:9 AS [SAUL/PAUL] TURNED AROUND TO LEAVE SAMUEL, GOD GAVE HIM ANOTHER HEART; AND ALL THOSE SIGNS WERE FULFILLED THAT SAME DAY.

Sadly there are not many who understand repentance because they do not recognize the LORD, so their only alternative is surgery and the probability that the doctor doesn't know the LORD is more common than we care to admit. Therefore it becomes a situation of the spiritually "dead" assisting the contaminated because the existent spiritual state of being of all unsaved persons is anesthetized[dead].

EPHESIANS 2:5 BUT GOD IS SO RICH IN MERCY AND LOVES US WITH SUCH INTENSE LOVE :5 THAT, EVEN WHEN WE

WERE DEAD BECAUSE OF OUR ACTS OF DISOBEDIENCE, HE BROUGHT US TO LIFE ALONG WITH THE MESSIAH, IT IS BY GRACE THAT YOU HAVE BEEN DELIVERED. JEWISH NEW TESTAMENT

The root cause of all problem is sin and if we righteously desire to lift the enslavement that iniquity causes we must repent, seek GOD and commence to place our sin beneath the Blood of YESHUA so that we may be divinely protected and hearty from the preventive rather than the curative.

Prescription drugs are founded in and rooted from poison that usually does not cure but can only dull the pain and often causes side effects that in due time will tarnish additional regions of our person. We would be prudent to pursue the natural curative or prevention and it is spelled 'Y-E-S-H-U-A' WHO was perfect in all HIS ways.

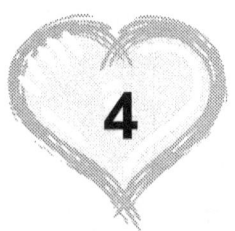

PREVENTATIVE HEALTH

If we consider the preventive we will remember thinking good and pure thoughts and feeding our mind and body on good and pure habits and food will naturally produce good health and pure thoughts.

The alternative to good is bad or evil, so to think on or feed our mind and body with evil will bring dis-ease to our body that GOD created to reject evil, consequently our body will begin to turn hard and callous. Thus causing hardening of the HEART, arteries, veins, etc.

ROMANS 2:3 DO YOU THINK THAT YOU, A MERE MAN PASSING JUDGMENT ON OTHERS WHO DO SUCH THINGS, YET DOING THEM YOURSELF, WILL ESCAPE THE JUDGMENT OF GOD? :4 OR PERHAPS YOU DESPISE THE RICHES OF HIS KINDNESS, FORBEARANCE AND PATIENCE; BECAUSE YOU DON'T REALIZE THAT GOD'S KINDNESS IS INTENDED TO LEAD YOU TO TURN FROM YOUR SINS. :5 BUT BY YOUR STUBBORNNESS, BY YOUR

UNREPENTANT HEART, YOU ARE STORING UP ANGER FOR YOURSELF ON THE DAY OF ANGER, WHEN GOD'S RIGHTEOUS JUDGMENT WILL BE REVEALED :6 FOR HE WILL PAY BACK EACH ONE ACCORDING TO HIS DEEDS :7 TO THOSE WHO SEEK GLORY, HONOR AND IMMORTALITY BY PERSEVERANCE IN DOING GOOD, HE WILL PAY BACK ETERNAL LIFE :8 BUT TO THOSE WHO ARE SELF-SEEKING, WHO DISOBEY THE TRUTH AND OBEY EVIL, HE WILL PAY BACK WRATH AND ANGER. JEWISH NEW TESTAMENT

The WORD of GOD is manna{food} from Heaven, angels diet for our spirit, what can be better?

Our thinking always affects our HEART first and if we manage the thoughts of our mind correctly we will make choices to have a happy HEART, which is a clean HEART free of anger, hate, bitterness, grudges and the like. It is a HEART that knows GOD and is balanced with the issues of life that affords wisdom and good understanding.

Our emotional and physical health are profitably to our well being and are closely related to our thoughts, so good thoughts will transcend any medicine and is the best reason to expect a healthy HEART. When we seek the higher lift, within the frame work of GOD'S Divine purpose we will be raised up by seeking GOD and lifted us to higher ground, above the greed, hate, and selfishness of our worldly surroundings.

A health preventive is always better than the curative and healthy thoughts will serve both because right thinking will prevent and/or correct troubles. MARCUE AURELIUS SAID 'A MAN'S LIFE IS WHAT HIS THOUGHTS MAKE IT'.

1 PETER 3:10 WHOEVER WANTS TO LOVE LIFE AND SEE GOOD DAYS MUST KEEP HIS TONGUE FROM EVIL AND HIS LIPS FROM SPEAKING DECEIT, :11 TURN FROM EVIL AND DO GOOD, SEEK PEACE AND CHASE AFTER IT :12 FOR ADONAI {THE LORD} KEEPS HIS EYES ON THE

RIGHTEOUS, AND HIS EARS ARE OPEN TO THEIR PRAYERS; BUT THE FACE OF ADONAI IS AGAINST THOSE WHO DO EVIL THINGS. JEWISH NEW TESTAMENT

This world is moving fast, days are chasing days never to catch up, only to die as another sunset turns yesterday into a fleeting memory. A moment we can never regain or change. How our days turn out depends on what we choose to put into them, for our days are products of our own creation but our power does not reach back or forward to change GOD'S plan. We need only to manage correctly the day we have, to spend it wisely.

While we are unmindful of outside forces which may present trials that will be helpful or hurtful to make our days good or bad by our reaction to those experiences. We are the pilot of our ship and it is not the wind, but the set of the sails {our thoughts} and the stirring of the rudder {our actions} that determine our direction.

We need to set up sails in our HEART and keep the rudder controlled by good and positive thoughts and ideas that spell health. To write {memorize} portion of GOD'S WORD on our HEART that speaks to us for instant recall so that when storm clouds gather or darken horizons we are competent to 'DRAW FROM THE WELL' of enthusiasm and vigor by speaking THE COMMANDMENTS from the WORD that can move mountains of despair, given by the only mountain mover that exist, WHO is, 'GOD'!

We must learn and be aware that fear, anger, fright, bitterness, anxiety, and the like are evil spirits meant for our defeat and only GOD can control them. But, if we don't know GOD we are without help and guidance.

The individual who will not stand for right, stands for nothing and will submit to anything. Subjecting themselves their children, grand children and loved ones to the exposure of misfortune and inflamed tribulations from the enemy which concludes our softness or hardness, for the same fire that hardens the clay melts the tallow.

For a contented life we need a right purpose, virtuous design and moral determination set daily within us that will put meaning into each day. With no direction the damper of mediocrity presents a deceptive danger that dwells outside the HEARTS door. This subtle enemy manifest through thoughts of status quo, rather than seeking GOD'S perfect will. Mediocrity and status quo spells death to GOD'S Divine destiny in life but when we put our HEART into a worthy work and travel in the direction of that goal we will find encouragement and great peace in the accomplishment. Precept upon precept, goal upon goal will cause our life to be full and at life's end we will be enthusiastic about passing into eternity and will have made loved ones proud to have been a part of our lives.

When we embrace GOD'S Wisdom, we will be overwhelmed by HIS marvelous mercy and love toward us, our energy and enthusiasm will make our lives invigorating, happy and healthy. Our thoughts will be preparing the way for the measure of a man lives with in his thoughts. By right living in GOD'S WILL and favor we build great treasure in eternity where the streets are gold and all is perfect.

2 CORINTHIANS 10:4 THE WEAPONS WE USE TO WAGE WAR ARE NOT WORLDLY. ON THE CONTRARY, THEY HAVE GOD'S POWER FOR DEMOLISHING STRONGHOLDS. WE DEMOLISH ARGUMENTS :5 AND EVERY ARROGANCE THAT RAISES ITSELF UP AGAINST THE KNOWLEDGE OF GOD; WE TAKE EVERY THOUGHT CAPTIVE AND MAKE IT OBEY THE MESSIAH :6 AND WHEN YOU HAVE BECOME COMPLETELY OBEDIENT, THEN WE WILL BE READY TO PUNISH EVERY ACT OF DISOBEDIENCE. JEWISH NEW TESTAMENT

Life is a mixture of sunshine and storms, encouragement and discouragement's, joys and sorrows and each has its accompanying effects upon our spirit. These effects are called moods, their temperament or mental veins influence all aspects of life, health and happiness, security and success. It is our duty to keep a hopeful, valiant and victorious disposition lest we assign many precious days of our fleeting lives to growing tension, gathering gloom and multiplying morbidity.

Those who look high in their expectations must aim high in those endeavors, and study to do the works of GOD, distinguished from the works of men in their worldly pursuits. It is not enough to speak the WORDS of GOD, we must do the Works of GOD. The work of faith is the industry of GOD and as our faith grows so to will our good works inspired by the HOLY SPIRIT, we will be empowered unto GOD'S Will in the home as well as in the streets.

GOD'S greatest desire is for our obedience to HIM, not for the sake of deception or conceit but that we reflect HIM and further HIS Kingdom to make it better known to all men by our Godly countenance, agape love and service to others. Yet with caution not to become arrogant or haughty for the HEART of one can discern the HEART of another and will sense truth or self-righteousness, compassion or pride. Our HEART disposition will determine anothers acceptance or rejection of our words.

If obedience and comfort follow the same path, GOD is pleased. But if the paths separate and obedience goes to the right while comfort goes to the left, we must choose the right and forsake comfort to stay in GOD'S Will.

Many well meaning men and pastors were called to GODLY vocation but fear came and faith left and they were found in unbelief, without faith and they could not stand. They chose the favor of men to stay comfortable and allowed fear to paralyze GOD'S Will in their lives.

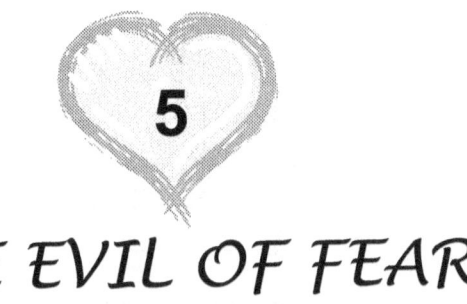

THE EVIL OF FEAR

Fear is imposed by satan that is only an evil spirit, but that tempter can be resisted with great force when we belong to GOD, for satan's only fear is GOD.

1 TIMOTHY 1:7 FOR GOD HATH NOT GIVEN US THE SPIRIT OF FEAR; BUT OF POWER, AND OF LOVE AND OF A SOUND MIND.

Even so we can not afford to ignore the spirit of fear or the effect it has in our life for it is a deadly bondage and if we allow it in any form even the apprehension will cause spiritual paralysis. The dread of fear will chain and cripple us and will drag us into the pits of hell eternally 'FOR WE ARE HELD BY THE CORDS OF OUR SIN' and bondage to fear is sin.

Psychologists say we are born with two fears. One of falling and the other of noise. But as we grow so does our fear, in fact this present age is frantic with fear.

Negative peer pressure swims and flourishes in fear and eventually erodes the pioneer spirit of GOD. It is a killer of destinies that will choke out any life if we do not know our authority we have as GOD'S Children.

Unbelief and doubt are synonymous with dread, alarm, fright, terror, apprehension, anxiety, perplexity, distrust and is known as fear.

There is victory and freedom in YESHUA and HE paid the price to deliver us from anxiety and fear but if we do not know HIM, that manifestation can not be a reality.

PSALMS 91:5 THOU SHALT NOT BE AFRAID FOR THE TERROR BY NIGHT, NOR FOR THE ARROW THAT FLIETH BY DAY. :6 NOR FOR THE PESTILENCE THAT WALKETH IN DARKNESS; NOR FOR THE DESTRUCTION THAT WASTETH AT NOONDAY. JEWISH TANAKH

Looking both ways before we cross the street or taking a vaccine to avoid polio are normal and good fears and should not be confused with cautions of unnecessary fright.

Deliverance from fear is one of GOD'S promises along with the inevitable and assured success that is ours when we make a conscience decision to surrender to HIS WILL for HE can not lie.

Our responsibilities are granted according to our abilities. It is our charge to do the best we can with a clean and earnest HEART and leave the results in the Hands of GOD, if we seek GOD HE will take all fear from our HEART and replace it with joy and courage even in the midst of the storm or the valley of the shadow of death.

PSALMS 23:4 THOUGH I WALK THROUGH A VALLEY OF DEEPEST DARKNESS, I FEAR NO HARM, FOR YOU ARE WITH ME; YOUR ROD AND YOUR STAFF- THEY COMFORT ME. JEWISH TANAKH

When we allow fright to take hold in our HEART it will operate with failure in mind. Our tendency will be to dread the unknown future, responsibility, old age, insecurity, growth, what others say and think about us and any thing that represents a stand against us. If we do not resist him satan will inundate us with technicalities of panic. GOD says:

JAMES 4:6 BUT THE GRACE HE GIVES IS GREATER, WHICH IS WHY IT SAYS, GOD OPPOSES THE ARROGANT, BUT TO THE HUMBLE HE GIVES GRACE :7 THEREFORE, SUBMIT TO GOD. MOREOVER, TAKE A STAND AGAINST THE adversary{satan}, AND HE WILL FLEE FROM YOU. JEWISH NEW TESTAMENT

The apprehension of fear will make life a wretched experience and warp the personality. It will prevent us from doing the Will of GOD and make us terrified of being known as a fanatic. It will render us useless and bring defeat for he who fears being conquered is sure of defeat.

Fear is an evil spirit that will bring on the very thing we fear most and it will spread, paralyze, kill and destroy but only if we allow it and refuse to claim GOD'S authority to rebuke and resist it.

Suicide has become the 10th ranking cause of death in our nation. Some 20,000 commit suicide each year. One young lady who had attempted suicide, when asked why she wanted to die, replied, "I was afraid to go on living".

GOD tells us approximately 180 times in HIS WORD not to fear for it is a characteristic of the wicked:

PROVERBS 28:1 THE WICKED FLEE WHERE NO MAN PURSUETH BUT THE RIGHTEOUS ARE BOLD AS A LION.

The dreaded fear of disease often brings on illness. In fact we are told that 85% of the emotional and physical ills of men are brought on by fear. The unsaved will always dread the horror of dying and that creates chains of bondage.

HEBREWS 2:15 THUS SET FREE THOSE WHO HAD BEEN IN BONDAGE ALL THEIR LIVES BECAUSE OF THEIR FEAR OF DEATH. JEWISH NEW TESTAMENT

With YESHUA enthroned in our HEARTS we need not fear, for to live is YESHUA and to die is gain and is pondered with joy because we will be with our Heavenly FATHER to live forevermore.

Courage is the opposite of fear and fear is eradicated by the consciousness of the LORD'S presence.

HEBREWS 13:6 SO THAT WE MAY BOLDLY SAY, THE LORD IS MY HELPER, AND I WILL NOT FEAR WHAT MAN SHALL DO UNTO ME.

Faith is a foe of fear and as long as we walk with the FATHER we can be confident and assured of our path since GOD the FATHER sends HIS ANGELS out before us to prepare our way and keep us in full assurance, knowing HE is with us simply because of our faith. Sin and fear are inseparable and satan manages and sends out both for our destruction.

PSALMS 34:16 THE EYES OF THE LORD ARE ON THE RIGHTEOUS, HIS EARS ATTENTIVE TO THEIR CRY. JEWISH TANAKH

Fear is usually fabricated due to a sense of guilt hidden in the HEART and for us to rid ourselves of guiltiness we must submit, repent and ask GOD to cleanse our HEART and renew HIS Spirit with in us. {PSALMS 51:10}

Heaven knows we need never be ashamed of our tears, for they are rain upon the blinding dust of earth, overlying our hard hearts. By: Charles Dickens

MATTHEW 10:28 DO NOT FEAR THOSE WHO KILL THE BODY BUT ARE POWERLESS TO KILL THE SOUL. RATHER,

FEAR HIM WHO CAN DESTROY BOTH SOUL AND BODY IN GEY-HINNOM {hell}. JEWISH NEW TESTAMENT

Reverential fear of GOD, is a controlling motive of life, in matters spiritual and moral, not a mere fear of HIS power and righteous retribution, but a wholesome dread of displeasing HIM, a fear which banishes the very terror that shrinks from HIS presence.

ROMANS 8:14 ALL WHO ARE LED BY GOD'S SPIRIT ARE GOD'S SONS :15 FOR YOU DID NOT RECEIVE A SPIRIT OF SLAVERY TO BRING YOU BACK AGAIN INTO FEAR; ON THE CONTRARY, YOU RECEIVED THE SPIRIT, WHO MAKES US SONS AND BY WHOSE POWER WE CRY OUT, "ABBA" {DEAR FATHER}} :16 THE SPIRIT HIMSELF BEARS WITNESS WITH OUR OWN SPIRITS THAT WE ARE CHILDREN OF GOD :17 AND IF WE ARE CHILDREN, THEN WE ARE ALSO HEIRS, HEIRS OF GOD AND JOINT-HEIRS WITH THE MESSIAH, PROVIDED WE ARE SUFFERING WITH HIM IN ORDER ALSO TO BE GLORIFIED WITH HIM. JEWISH NEW TESTAMENT

GOD'S presence will always influence the disposition and attitude of our circumstances and are guided by our trust in HIM through HIS indwelling HOLY SPIRIT. Most of our fears relate either to the past or the future and we need to remember that the past is a spent check and the future is a promissory note. Only our present is ready cash and we must spend it wisely without fear or worry.

We must learn to love the neighbor, the store keeper, the stranger as well as members of our family regardless of what they do that hurt or offend us. The key is love, because love covers a multitude of sin and we will find that the more we love, the less we fear and the easier it becomes to find reason to overcome our fear. Our HEART will be focused on someone else besides 'self' and we will find it easy to forget our woes, the big "I" we surround ourselves with will have deminished. It has often been said that it is better to have loved and lost than never have loved at all.

1 PETER 4:8 MORE THAN ANYTHING, KEEP LOVING EACH OTHER ACTIVELY; BECAUSE LOVE COVERS MAN SINS. JEWISH NEW TESTAMENT

PRIDE AND ARROGANCE

Guard against pride for it was pride and arrogance that destroyed Lucifer and caused GOD to damn him{satan} to hell for eternity and it will destroy any who adhere to its lift to wear it on the cuff.

1 CORINTHIANS 8:1b 'WE ALL HAVE KNOWLEDGE, YES, THAT IS SO, BUT KNOWLEDGE PUFFS UP WITH PRIDE; WHEREAS LOVE BUILDS UP.

When we put down pride and pick up love we will heal the differences of denominations and racism as well as those who walk among and beside us, we must remember that those who feel and look different may also be a part of the BODY and we are never to think we are the only chosen people or no one else is as good or able to please YESHUA or belong to HIM for that attitude is smothered in pride. The doctrine which is according to GODLINESS, is that which is productive of GODLINESS. The mystery of GODLINESS is embodied in and communicated through the truths of the faith concerning YESHUA.

MARK 10:18 YESHUA SAID TO HIM, WHY ARE YOU CALLING ME GOOD? NO ONE IS GOOD EXCEPT GOD. JEWISH NEW TESTAMENT

When we depend upon our own wisdom, we are in danger of being prideful and self-seeking and are indulging in idol worship of selfishness. That frame of mind works self righteousness and even YESHUA, WHO was found to be perfect in all HIS ways refused to allow others to glorify HIM and HE grieved that any would consider them selves above HIS HEAVENLY FATHER as HE said:

MATTHEW 19:17 WHY ARE YOU ASKING ME ABOUT GOOD? THERE IS ONE WHO IS GOOD! BUT IF YOU WANT TO OBTAIN ETERNAL LIFE OBSERVE THE MITZVOTH [COMMANDMENTS] JEWISH NEW TESTAMENT

We must be careful not to judge or be critical of others who profess to be part of HIS BODY but walk a different path. If we will look to the SCRIPTURE GOD often used mysterious people in strange and bizarre ways to perform or reach HIS goals and what is bizarre and abnormal to us might be customary for another. SCRIPTURE tells us:

ROMANS 15:4 FOR EVERYTHING WRITTEN IN THE PAST WAS WRITTEN TO TEACH US, SO THAT WITH THE ENCOURAGEMENT OF THE TANAKH/OLD TESTAMENT WE MIGHT PATIENTLY HOLD ON TO OUR HOPE :5 AND MAY GOD, THE SOURCE OF ENCOURAGEMENT AND PATIENCE, GIVE YOU THE SAME ATTITUDE AMONG YOURSELVES AS THE MESSIAH YESHUA HAD. JEWISH NEW TESTAMENT

"Look to this day, for it is life. In its brief course live all the verities and realities of your existence; the bliss of growth, the glory of action, the splendor of beauty. For yesterday is but a dream, and tomorrow is only a vision; but today, well lived, makes every yesterday a dream of happiness and every tomorrow a vision of hope. Look well, therefore, to this day, such is the salvation of the dawn". - From the Sanscrit

Happiness can be found in the thoughts we choose to entertain. If we are wise to choose good and wholesome thoughts, we will find peace but if we choose evil, hateful, controlling, greedy thoughts we will find confusion and hell for the mind manages the thoughts we feed it and will be faithful to manifest the attitude we make up our mind to cherish. We must guard our eyes from seeing evil that will penetrate our minds and enter our HEART for evil is destruction and if we follow evil we will never be able to say I can and I will just as Paul said in:

PHILIPPINES 4:13 "I CAN DO ALL THINGS THROUGH YESHUA WHICH STRENGTHENETH ME" JEWISH NEW TESTAMENT

Paul chose to submit to YESHUA and seek the Will of GOD because he knew there was no challenge or burden to difficult for him to handle with the LORD'S help. His HEART was confident of the victory of an unconquerable spirit and heroic life.

No man is beaten unless his thoughts are beaten and he can not falter as long as he knows and submits to GOD where all unique strength comes from. We must seek THE WORD daily for spiritual feeding for the sharpened Sword of HIS Spirit within us is the reason we win the battle. Only HIS WORD can whittle our self-righteous importance to a distinct effectiveness that is useable for GOD.

THE BATTLEFIELD is between GOD and the devil and it began when the devil lifted himself up in pride but our victory was completed as GOD sent HIS ONLY SON YESHUA WHO freely gave HIS life as a Lamb to Slaughter at Golgotha {Calvary}.

The record of YESHUA'S{JESUS}Sacrificial death is given in the first four Gospels of the Church Covenant {New Testament} and are Prophesy fulfilled from the Jewish Covenant {Old Testament}.

One wonders how such a thing could happen? Was not the MESSIAH GOD incarnate? Indeed HE was! How, then, could GOD have actually died on the cross? Lets return to Genesis where Adam was created and his tragic sin. GOD had warned him that disobedience would result in death, and so it did. In fact, it brought down upon the head of mankind two kinds of death: physical and spiritual. Both kinds of death here can be defined by one word, separation. That is the biblical and theological meaning of the word death. Physical death is separation, the parting of the soul from one's body. Spiritual death is likewise separation, the parting of the unsaved person from GOD. This is some times called the second death.

REVELATION 20:14 THEN DEATH AND SH'OL {HELL} WERE HURLED INTO THE LAKE OF FIRE. THIS IS THE SECOND DEATH, THE LAKE OF FIRE. :15 ANYONE WHOSE NAME WAS NOT FOUND WRITTEN IN THE BOOK OF LIFE WAS HURLED INTO THE LAKE OF FIRE. JEWISH NEW TESTAMENT

Physical and spiritual death are two hellish enemies let loose by Adam and continued to curse and terrorize the human race for over forty centuries. Then in the fullness of time, GOD sent HIS beloved SON to this world and referred to HIM as the last Adam.

1 CORINTHIANS 15:45 IN FACT, THE TANAKH SAYS SO: ADAM, THE FIRST MAN, BECAME A LIVING HUMAN BEING; BUT THE LAST 'ADAM' HAS BECOME A LIFE GIVING SPIRIT. JEWISH NEW TESTAMENT

The Second Adam had come to undo what the first Adam had previously done; HE came to rid mankind of those two evil enemies, physical and spiritual death. This HE did while on the cross, where HE died spiritually, being separated from GOD; and died physically as HE accomplished both tasks. Spiritual death was immediately given the death blow. Paul later assured us that nothing could separate us from the love of GOD

ROMANS 8:35 WHO WILL SEPARATE US FROM THE LOVE OF THE MESSIAH? TROUBLE? HARDSHIP? PERSECUTION? HUNGER? POVERTY? DANGER? WAR? :36 AS THE TANAKH PUTS IT, "FOR YOUR SAKE WE ARE BEING PUT TO DEATH ALL DAY LONG, WE ARE CONSIDERED SHEEP TO BE SLAUGHTERED. PSALMS 44:23" :37 NO, IN ALL THESE THINGS WE ARE SUPER CONQUERORS, THROUGH THE ONE WHO HAS LOVED US. :38 FOR I AM CONVINCED THAT NEITHER DEATH NOR LIFE, NEITHER ANGELS NOR OTHER HEAVENLY RULERS, NEITHER WHAT EXISTS NOR WHAT IS COMING :39 NEITHER POWERS ABOVE NOR POWERS BELOW, NOR ANY OTHER CREATED THING WILL BE ABLE TO SEPARATE US FROM THE LOVE OF GOD WHICH COME TO US THROUGH THE MESSIAH YESHUA {JESUS}, OUR LORD. JEWISH NEW TESTAMENT

BUT WHAT ABOUT PHYSICAL DEATH? PAUL ANSWERS THAT IN:

1 CORINTHIANS 15:51 LOOK, I WILL TELL YOU A SECRET, NOT ALL OF US WILL DIE! BUT WE WILL ALL BE CHANGED! :52 IT WILL TAKE BUT A MOMENT, THE BLINK OF AN EYE, AT THE FINAL SHOFAR {TRUMPET}. FOR THE SHOFAR {TRUMPET} WILL SOUND, AND THE DEAD WILL BE RAISED TO LIVE FOREVER, AND WE TOO WILL BE CHANGED. :53 FOR THIS MATERIAL WHICH CAN DECAY MUST BE CLOTHED WITH IMPERISHABILITY, THIS WHICH IS MORTAL MUST BE CLOTHED WITH IMMORTALITY. :54 WHEN WHAT DECAYS PUTS ON IMPERISHABILITY AND

WHAT IS MORTAL PUTS ON IMMORTALITY, THEN THIS PASSAGE IN THE TANAKH WILL BE FULFILLED; "DEATH IS SWALLOWED BY IN VICTORY. ISAIAH 25:8" :55 "DEATH, WHERE IS YOUR VICTORY? DEATH, WHERE IS YOUR STING. HOSEA 13:14" :56 THE STING OF DEATH IS SIN; AND SIN DRAWS ITS POWER FROM THE TORAH; :57 BUT THANKS BE TO GOD, WHO GIVES US THE VICTORY THROUGH OUR LORD YESHUA {JESUS} THE MESSIAH! :58 SO, MY DEAR BROTHERS STAND FIRM AND UNMOVABLE, ALWAYS DOING THE LORD'S WORK AS VIGOROUSLY AS YOU CAN, KNOWING THAT UNITED WITH THE LORD YOUR EFFORTS ARE NOT IN VAIN. JEWISH NEW TESTAMENT

YESHUA was crucified at Golgotha which is commonly known as the skull, {place of the mind}.

Even though we were created for GOD'S pleasure we are restrained here on earth and given free will to make a conscience choice of which GOD or god we will serve. We are caught in the mist of this battle between GOD and satan and satan, the accuser always begins with the mind. GOD had preordained YESHUA'S crucifixion, even though satan thought the defeat and death of YESHUA would make him the master. Thus the great impostor was deceived when YESHUA went into the dregs of hell to take the keys to death and the grave from the devil.

MATTHEW 20:28 FOR THE SON OF MAN DID NOT COME TO BE SERVED, BUT TO SERVE AND TO GIVE HIS LIFE AS A RANSOM FOR MANY. JEWISH NEW TESTAMENT

Old Covenant prophecy was fulfilled as YESHUA was raised from the dead. HE was seen by more than 500 persons before HE ascended into Heaven to set upon the right hand of GOD the FATHER.

MARK 14:62 "I AM," ANSWERED YESHUA. MOREOVER, YOU WILL SEE THE SON OF MAN SITTING AT THE RIGHT HAND

OF HAG'VURAH {THE POWER;i.e., GOD} AND COMING ON THE CLOUDS OF HEAVEN. JEWISH NEW TESTAMENT

The mind {skull} is ceaselessly satan's target and he slams the human mind repeatedly with evil poisonous darts of deception. However the devil is powerless to pass through the BLOOD of YESHUA and YESHUA'S BLOOD is our "only" defense even so the option of who we obey is ours and it equals to serving evil and being tormented, cursed and destroyed or staying armed with YESHUA'S WORD, covered by HIS BLOOD and up holding HIS STANDARDS in the face of evil. The believer is never told to attack the devil, but to withstand and resist him.

1 PETER 5:8 STAY SOBER, STAY ALERT! YOUR enemy, THE adversary, STALKS ABOUT LIKE A ROARING LION LOOKING FOR SOMEONE TO DEVOUR. :9 STAND AGAINST him FIRM IN YOUR TRUST, KNOWING THAT YOUR BROTHERS THROUGH OUT THE WORLD ARE GONG THROUGH THE SAME KINDS OF SUFFERING. JEWISH NEW TESTAMENT

It is those who submit to YESHUA with the whole HEART that are under the divine covering and protection of the Precious and perfect BLOOD of YESHUA and who have authority in HIM to resist satan and 'he must flee'.

When we assume a rational portrayal of ourselves as saved by the BLOOD of YESHUA we have moved forward to know that we are capable, cheerful, likable, and dynamic and that our mental image will develop into an actual relationship with the LORD. Healthy thinking will produce healthy feelings therefore we must practice affirming good and pleasant forecasts, as we learn to count our blessings we will successfully cast off negative thoughts.

COLOSSIANS 3:14 ABOVE ALL THESE, CLOTHE YOURSELVES WITH LOVE, WHICH BINDS EVERYTHING TOGETHER PERFECTLY; :15 AND LET THE SHALOM {PEACE} WHICH

COMES FROM THE MESSIAH BE YOUR HEART'S DECISION-MAKER, FOR THIS IS WHY YOU WERE CALLED TO BE PART OF A SINGLE BODY. AND BE THANKFUL :16 LET THE WORD OF THE MESSIAH, IN ALL ITS RICHNESS, LIVE IN YOU, AS YOU TEACH AND COUNSEL EACH OTHER IN ALL WISDOM AND AS YOU SING PSALMS, HYMNS AND SPIRITUAL SONGS WITH GRATITUDE TO GOD IN YOUR HEARTS. :17 THAT IS, EVERYTHING YOU DO OR SAY, DO IN THE NAME OF THE LORD YESHUA, GIVING THANKS THROUGH HIM TO GOD THE FATHER. JEWISH NEW TESTAMENT

Gratitude and affirmation go together and we need to always be thankful nevertheless doubt is a negative power which will bring defeat, gloom, restlessness and wretched health to all who are victimized by it. It is a physio-logically accepted fact that when faith breaks down, the nervous system often times does too. To be called of GOD is a great honor and if we pursue it GOD will exalt us but man will crucify us. The battle is to be and remain faithful.

GOD CALLS. GOD'S call to the disciples was a divine decree, not a sweet suggestion. There was no option just as there is no options for us. If we want a good healthy HEART we will be wise to listen, heed and follow HIS will when GOD calls us to service. GOD doesn't promise profit sharing, stock options, retirement plans, fringe benefits, a rose garden or other perks. Often there will be no position of importance among men, no board meetings to talk about raising money, building new buildings or developing new programs or gimmicks to build people numbers for donations.

The call begins with long hours on the knees, grieving for the salvation of others, praying for the unloved, lost, undone and sick, our HEART will not desire to do other wise. These tactics will build mansions in Heaven for all of eternity and the short time spent here can't to be compared to forever and forever and forever in eternity.

EPHESIANS 1:7 IN UNION WITH HIM, THROUGH THE SHEDDING OF HIS BLOOD, WE ARE SET FREE, OUR SINS ARE FORGIVEN; THIS ACCORDS WITH THE WEALTH OF THE GRACE :8 HE HAS LAVISHED ON US. IN ALL HIS WISDOM AND INSIGHT :9 HE HAS MADE KNOWN TO US HIS SECRET PLAN, WHICH BY HIS OWN WILL HE DESIGNED BEFOREHAND IN CONNECTION WITH THE MESSIAH :10 AND WILL PUT INTO EFFECT WHEN THE TIME IS RIPE, HIS PLAN TO PLACE EVERYTHING IN HEAVEN AND ON EARTH UNDER THE MESSIAH'S HEADSHIP.   JEWISH NEW TESTAMENT

Our eternity is not determined in a court of men or judged by peers but by the MASTER CREATOR. It is a matter of the HEART and if we are poured out before HIM, HE will fill us with HIS SPIRIT. Our teardrops for others will be molded into precious pearls by GOD, WHO is pleased to reserve and weave them into crowns of magnificent glory for our homecoming.

As long as we walk in flesh, we are grounded in a combat zone but when we are protected by HIS Armor {EPH. 6} we stand in readiness for the battle with the SWORD of HIS SPIRIT which is identified with the WORD OF GOD.

EPHESIANS 6:10 FINALLY GROW POWERFUL IN UNION WITH THE LORD, IN UNION WITH HIS MIGHTY STRENGTH! :11 USE ALL THE ARMOR AND WEAPONRY THAT GOD PROVIDES, SO THAT YOU WILL BE ABLE TO STAND AGAINST THE DECEPTIVE TACTICS OF THE ADVERSARY. :12 FOR WE ARE NOT STRUGGLING AGAINST HUMAN BEINGS, BUT AGAINST THE RULERS, AUTHORITIES AND COSMIC POWERS GOVERNING THIS DARKNESS, AGAINST THE SPIRITUAL FORCES OF EVIL IN

THE HEAVENLY REALM. :13 SO TAKE UP EVERY PIECE OF WAR EQUIPMENT GOD PROVIDES; SO THAT WHEN THE EVIL DAY COMES, YOU WILL STILL BE STANDING. :14 THEREFORE, STAND! HAVE THE BELT OF TRUTH BUCKLED AROUND YOUR WAIST, PUT ON RIGHTEOUSNESS FOR A BREASTPLATE. :15 AND WEAR ON YOUR FEET THE READINESS THAT COMES FROM THE GOOD NEWS OF SHALOM {PEACE} :16 ALWAYS CARRY THE SHIELD OF TRUST, WITH WHICH YOU WILL BE ABLE TO EXTINGUISH ALL THE FLAMING ARROWS OF THE EVIL ONE :17 AND TAKE THE HELMET OF DELIVERANCE; ALONG WITH THE SWORD GIVEN BY THE SPIRIT, THAT IS, THE WORLD OF GOD; :18 AS YOU PRAY AT ALL TIMES, WITH ALL KINDS OF PRAYERS AND REQUESTS. IN THE SPIRIT, VIGILANTLY AND PERSISTENTLY, FOR ALL GOD'S PEOPLE. JEWISH NEW TESTAMENT

1. Principalities are believed to be satan's generals
2. Powers believed to be privates who possess humans
3. World rulers thought to be demons in charge of worldly business
4. Spiritual wickedness believed to be demons in charge of worldly religion
5. Wiles of the devil refers to cunning arts, deceit, craft, trickery. 1 Tim 3:7; 2 Cor 2:11
6. Firey darts of wiles are arrows tipped with tow, pitch or the like and set fire and discharged toward believers
7. Truth - A believer whose life is tainted with deceit and falsehood forfeits the very thing that holds other pieces of GOD's Armor together.
8. Breastplate of Righteousness speaks of right acts and is devised to protect the HEART of the soldier.

Thus un-righteous acts committed by a believer robs him of vital protection and exposes his spiritual HEART to satan.

9.	The Sandals are believed to be in reference to sure footing, assurance and confidence which come from knowing the great doctrinal truths associated with the Gospel.

10. Helmet of Salvation protects the head and brain and refers to the Study of the Gospel, keeping covered by GOD'S wisdom and Perfect Blood of the LAMB - YESHUA. SOURCE: WILMINGTON'S GUIDE TO THE BIBLE

With GOD we are fortified and refined, the tune in the HEART always controls the tone of our mental and physical state of health. We can be confident of our triumph because HE dispatches HIS supernatural beings to go before us to prepare our passage, to liquidate and eliminate the mountainous country that in our flesh and blood we could not oppose.

MARK 9:23 IF THOU CANST BELIEVE, ALL THINGS ARE POSSIBLE TO HIM THAT BELIEVETH. JEWISH NEW TESTAMENT

The meaningful emotional issues surrounding us have a tendency to become attached and effect our mental balance through expectation or anticipation and without GOD they are likely to provoke torment that will dwell in our spirit. They will cause our flesh to desire and gaze on harmful baggage that will tarnish our mental and physical state. Ungodly goods will spiritually execute THE HEART when we embrace them.

Tragically most humans are pessimistic and reflective thinkers, consequently these attitudes will harvest within the flesh and produce crippling, defeating effects such as weakness, dread, depreciation, depression, failure, disease or decrepitude. Without warning we rise up to profess and express sorrow for our dilemma, thus we generate their possessions to promote bodily ills as we gather and hide these matters in our sub-conscious {the dark corners of our mind}.

GOD is Holy and HE has given to HIS children holiness and moral conditions necessary for our health. When we walk in HIS Holiness we become healthy because HE is health. This is not an outward Holiness but inward. Our thoughts control us and as we think on GOD we are drawn nearer to HIM and HIS intended purpose for our life and HE bestows HIS SPIRIT on us justly and freely.

1 CORINTHIANS 13:1 I MAY SPEAK IN THE TONGUES OF MEN, EVEN ANGELS; BUT IF I LACK LOVE, I HAVE BECOME MERELY BLARING BRASS OR A CYMBAL CLANGING. :2 I MAY HAVE THE GIFT OF PROPHECY, I MAY FATHOM ALL MYSTERIES, KNOW ALL THINGS, HAVE ALL FAITH, ENOUGH TOMOVE MOUNTAINS; BUT IF I LACK LOVE I AM NOTHING. :3 I MAY GIVE AWAY EVERYTHING I OWN, I MAY EVEN HAND OVER MY BODY TO BE BURNED; BUT IF I LACK LOVE I GAIN NOTHING. :4 LOVE IS PATIENT AND KIND, NOT JEALOUS, NOT BOASTFUL, :5 NOT PROUD, RUDE OR SELFISH, NOT EASILY ANGERED, AND IT KEEPS NO RECORD OF WRONGS. :6 LOVE DOES NOT GLOAT OVER OTHER PEOPLE'S SIN BUT TAKES ITS DELIGHT IN THE TRUTH :7 LOVE ALWAYS BEARS UP, ALWAYS TRUSTS, ALWAYS HOPES, ALWAYS ENDURES. :8 LOVE NEVER ENDS; BUT PROPHECIES WILL PASS, TONGUES WILL CEASE, KNOWLEDGE WILL PASS. :9 FOR OUR KNOWLEDGE IS PARTIAL, AND OUR PROPHECY PARTIAL; :10 BUT WHEN THE PERFECT COMES, THE PARTIAL WILL PASS. :11 WHEN I WAS A CHILD I SPOKE LIKE A CHILD, THOUGHT LIKE A CHILD, ARGUED LIKE A CHILD; NOW THAT I HAVE BECOME A MAN, I HAVE FINISHED WITH CHILDISH WAYS. :12 FOR NOW WE SEE OBSCURELY IN A MIRROR, BUT THEN IT WILL BE FACE TO FACE. NOW I KNOW PARTLY; THEN I WILL KNOW FULLY, JUST AS GOD HAS FULLY KNOWN ME. :13 BUT FOR NOW, THREE THINGS

LAST, TRUST, HOPE, LOVE AND THE GREATEST OF THESE IS LOVE! PURSUE LOVE.   JEWISH NEW TESTAMENT

WE must discern and be alert to scrutinize everything we tolerate to infringe our vision and mind because the HEART is a VITAL ORGAN that has a tendency to establish security barriers for keeping out encumbrances we want to escape from and worshipping the baggage that we lust to cleave too. As the guard rails go up they develop attitudes that will conceal a hopeless declaration of dread and distress and we will draw away from others into self. In our panic and chaos we attract self pity unless we have an exclusive alliance with CHRIST and understand HE is our defense.

Many of us have witnessed HIS phenomenal forgiveness and commitment but in disregard or unbelief we refuse to seek the MESSIAH until we suddenly arrive at the end of ourselves. Even so, GOD in HIS Divine compassion will answer in whatever place we are, HE will meet us in the depths to promote us, make us pure and collect us as HIS OWN if we will only repent from the HEART. But if the HEART institutes rejection of HIS WORD {YESHUA} it will entrap the soul in the dungeon of the enemy and we will become held by strongholds that will prevent and choke our livelihood thus we will suffer judgment and death.

As long as we reject YESHUA {JESUS-SON of GOD} we will trudge in ignorance. Our limits will introduce irritation to our character that was designed to radiate GOD'S plan, to opus with others and to overlook imperfections. To forgive others as GOD has pardoned us.

The corruption and dis-ease of resistance will either generate ailments or it will purify us for GOD'S Work, depending upon the sensibility of our HEART. Right, like sweet cream has a way of rising to the top; while wrong, like spilled milk, wastes itself in useless absorption.

There is none today who has not experienced ill-treatment and suffering, no matter how affluent or destitute, none are immuned. Perhaps it is GOD'S way to keep us humble, to keep our arrogance in review so that we will understand that we have no greater authority or ability than our associates, without THE LORD.

There are many that grip a prejudice or affliction and permit it to trickle into the hush-hush cubbyholes of the mind and create pollution, it will camouflage itself only to appear later masked as bitterness and hostility. Such actions will always create a cancerous energy in the HEART. Concealed away without forewarning we become vindictive, fearful, resentful and frequently pride ourselves in heartache and agony as we become attached to and value poisonous self-worship. Yearning for others to sympathize with us usually in an attempt to manipulate them.

When evil, fright or inconvenience is embraced and acclaimed it invades our being, generating within the HEART it dictates and dominates the body to introduce a production of dis-ease that will usher in infection and eventually disease. The wretched disposition is reflected to the world and pleads to be enjoined by whining to others and those we love often expecting their full attention.

Wrapped miserly in our own world of self pity attempting to make others feel responsible for our suffering, wounds or displeasure. Our dis-ease becomes contagious and transcends to those we rely on in diverse ways until it begins to mold our sickness, bitterness or pride, etc. on to them and the old adage of 'misery loves company' has conquered another. Is it any wonder that disease and sickness runs rampied in our society? We ignore GOD'S laws of health and wellness to do satan's unspeakable acts of death, and yet we wonder why so many are sick and dying? Blinded by the enemy of GOD and the killer of our soul.

There is nothing more offensive to GOD than a narrow, self-caring spirit. GOD refuses to be involved with or have any part in an evil work. HE will not recognize one who manifest the attributes of satan for they are insensible to the working of HIS SPIRIT and can not please HIM. They are evil works of unbelief and lack of faith.

The calamities that fall upon us are frequently caused from our attitude and unbelief and are often warnings from GOD as HE sharply rebukes our ignorance and indifference. The signs in the sky foretell the weather and we are quick to read them but the signs of the times, which so clearly point to HIS mission for our lives, are not discerned but rather ignored.

COMPASSION THROUGH HIS WORD

YESHUA'S calling is one of compassion in its alliance to GOD's impartiality and judicious reasoning and it is illustrated through out HIS WORD. In all things YESHUA said and did HE was aggressively assaulting the domination of corruption. When HE healed the sick, cast out evil spirit, preached the Gospel or made intercession for the people, HE was occupied in spiritual warfare.

When HE challenged the impious, self-righteous Pharisees in their powerless culture and outright sin HE was confronting satan himself. Unafraid of the consequences of suffering and death HIS mission in life was exhaustively utilized to fulfill HIS FATHER'S Will. The enslavement of sickness, disease and torment were demolished because of the anointing upon YESHUA.

1 JOHN 3:8 HE THAT COMMITTETH SIN IS OF THE DEVIL, FOR THE DEVIL SINNETH FROM THE BEGINNING. FOR

THIS PURPOSE THE SON OF GOD WAS MANIFESTED, THAT HE MIGHT DESTROY THE WORKS OF THE DEVIL.

The absolute incentive for YESHUA to visit earth was to manifest [become visible]to humankind as GOD'S WORD in flesh to cancel, become unbound, exterminate and destroy satan's enslavement. YESHUA'S assignment was prophesied and completed in the annihilation of the enemy at Calvary.

Nevertheless many are incapable of turning to GOD for lack of confidence or skepticism. In their destitution, torment and investigation for something to satisfy the emptiness of life they turn to the physic driven by satanic powers that will employ the intellect in amusement and create tribulation, thus in the end they are lured into eternal damnation for all eternity.

Psychic influence is called an abomination in THE WORD and has long been established that the telepathic medium has a decisive power in producing illness yet most of the world today has turned extravagantly to the psychics, chasing images from the mind and browsing the afterlife, unaware of the danger of the psychic network satan brings into being to steal, kill and destroy. The wizardry psychic's manage is a lying reflection set up by the monarch of hell to pervert, violate and lay a trap for those who are weak.

Consequently a physic is no more than a sorcerer, a wizard, a pretender of magic powers, a professor of the arts of witchcraft, a maker of horoscopes [lies from the pit of hell], a worker for satan, endowed with satan's powers to enslave and afflict us.

DEUT. 18:10 THERE SHALL NOT BE FOUND AMONG YOU ANYONE WHO MAKETH HIS SON OR HIS DAUGHTER PASS THROUGH THE FIRE {ABORTION}, OR WHO USETH DIVINATION OR AN OBSERVER OF TIMES {ASTROLOGY}, OR AN ENCHANTER {USER OF OMENS}, OR A WITCH {MAKES MAGIC} :11 OR A CHARMER, OR A CONSULTER OF MEDIUMS, OR A WIZARD, OR A NECROMANCER {SEEKS

USE OF THE DEAD}. :12 FOR ALL THAT DO THESE THINGS ARE AN ABOMINATION UNTO THE LORD; AND BECAUSE OF THESE ABOMINATIONS THE LORD THY GOD DOTH DRIVE THEM OUT FROM BEFORE THEE KJV

In Acts Shim'on went through the City practicing magic and astonishing all, claiming to be exalted but in-fact was a practicing magician who favored powers and controlling others. While his authority was supernatural it was never the less from hell. In Acts 8:18-23 Shim'on had fooled many as they followed him due to their own disbelief, choosing not GOD'S intelligence but satan's.

Today depraved spirits of Shim'on live and flourish in mortals who resolved themselves as one who sees into the future. But their insight and authority is received from the destructive one, GOD'S arch adversary, our assaulter lucifer who conjurers up magic that becomes a seduction into hell, taking pleasure from the attention for their illusive intuition which was born in the cavity of hell-fire. Even so GOD has left us with unwavering affirmations such as the ultimate destination of satan, his workers and works in:

REVELATION 21:8 BUT AS FOR THE COWARDLY, THE UNTRUSTWORTHY, THE VILE, THE MURDERERS, THE SEXUALLY IMMORAL, THOSE WHO MISUSE DRUGS IN CONNECTION WITH THE OCCULT, IDOL-WORSHIPPERS, AND ALL LIARS, THEIR DESTINY IS THE LAKE BURNING WITH FIRE AND SULFUR, THE SECOND DEATH.

Sorcery in the literal sense is witchcraft but as a wolf in sheep's clothing, it seeps in deliberately flowered in the witchery of lighthearted luxurious vice contaminated with sin as its attendant idolatries flood the minds eye with fascination and in that enlightened betrayal of the mind, and short-lived twinkling of festivity we are led astray in bewilderment to slaughter.

One of America's initial encounters with witch-craft was set up long ago through the TV sitcom, known as 'Bewitched' and as we set back in laughter to concentrate on one of America's delightful film celebrities twitch her adorable nose to bring about mischievous magical achievements of good or so called white witchcraft, we were lulled into a trance and seduced into demonology only to gain consciousness and find the prince of darkness had flourished and sorcery had become a standard turn of the mill, everyday celebration and everyone was gathering to approve the witch and her crafts.

Even though sorcery is a contemptible and destructive evil and those who ensue or pursue it are condemned to hell many of our every day dilemmas deliver hell into focus frequently as we yield to unforgiving attitudes, hatred, greed, and diverse hostile attitudes that GOD rebukes as they gain entry to take up residence in our life. Evil spirits that will root pain and push others away from us.

At a time when we most need someone to love and understand us, the evil spirits that have us bound within force those who care for us and whom we care most about to move further from us, causing grief, pain and questions of why, totally blinded by the enemy.

END TIMES

In the end each one will be judged by the CREATOR HIMSELF for what ever our style of life and where ever our grave. Our trial will be held for what we have approved of to happen or done in the brief life span on this planet according to what has been written in 'THE BOOK OF LIFE' which will stress undivided fairness of the examination.

The forum of justice may reflect the current court procedure but it will have every detail and trait cataloged through an elaborate spy system. Every jot and tittle will be provided by the MASTER, WHO is TRUTH DIVINE, WHO WILL NOT CHANGE AND CAN NOT LIE.

GOOD NEWS!! There is a path of escape that will project victory prepared exclusively for all who accept and follow YESHUA. Any other method of victory, salvation or eternal life is a fabrication prepared by the enemy to entice and seduce us into the pit of hell-fire. Thus it is mandatory for us to pursue GOD'S approval in all spheres of our mortality.

MATTHEW 6:33 BUT SEEK YE FIRST THE KINGDOM OF GOD, AND HIS RIGHTEOUSNESS, AND ALL THESE THINGS SHALL BE ADDED UNTO YOU.

The preceding verse is Heaven's unfailing blueprint for acquiring the essentials of life, to seek foremost GOD'S kingdom righteousness. This involves all the attributes associated with the nobler life such as faith, hope, love, dependence and diligence, work and thrift. It discounts laziness and irresponsibility for GOD'S way is not the way of the spendthrift or sluggard.

PROVERBS 6:6 GO TO THE ANT, THOU SLUGGARD; CONSIDER HER WAYS, AND BE WISE

The plenteous life can not be encountered by habitual idleness, waste, wrong thinking or wrong living. The full cupboard is only for those who will do their part to fill it.

We live in an spine tingling eye-popping era, a time when it is urgent for all who confess and belong to GOD'S family to awake, arise, fill the cupboard, challenge and engage the enemy in warfare to relinquish our territory. We are compelled to rescue our family as well as our state of health through spiritual warfare = prayer and righteous attitude.

The battlefield for our soul has been revealed and some have awakened to the cry of the HEART. Good days are found in good speech which bespeaks a good HEART; OUT OF THE ABUNDANCE OF THE HEART THE MOUTH SPEAKETH

MATTHEW 12:33 IF YOU MAKE A TREE GOOD, ITS FRUIT WILL BE GOOD; AND IF YOU MAKE A TREE BAD, ITS FRUIT WILL BE BAD; FOR A TREE IS KNOWN BY ITS FRUIT :34 YOU SNAKES! HOW CAN YOU WHO ARE EVIL SAY ANY THING GOOD? FOR THE MOUTH SPEAKS WHAT OVERFLOWS FROM THE HEART. JEWISH NEW TESTAMENT

The happy life requires the bridling of the tongue that could run loose and the sealing of lips that tend to utter guile if not properly managed. We are deceived if we think our tongue can not hurt others without also hurting us, so we should always refrain from speaking intolerant words, sarcastic utterances, adverse criticisms and wrathful outpourings.

"A WORD FILTHY SPOKEN" adds to fitting days and beautiful living "LIKE APPLES OF GOLD IN PICTURES OF SILVER".

The pleasant life in GOD'S WILL shuns ugliness and spreads pleasantries among others. We keep ourselves by keeping our brother. The world's shortest and sweetest biography tells of a life of concern and goodness for others

ACTS 10:38 "WHO WENT ABOUT DOING GOOD" THE STORY OF YESHUA.

When we truly know YESHUA from the HEART we will gainfully fulfill a mission to harmonize willingly with a desire to be a prepared people of destiny, eager to comply with GOD'S design. If we are unconcerned with that destiny we are in danger of spending our undivided existence in a state of perpetual wonderment. We will speculate aimlessly with no purpose or direction, no fire or zeal. The HOLY SPIRIT will have been quenched to set by in anticipation, waiting for the HEART to awaken but in our aimless perpetual tranquil state of mediocre we dare not step past the mediocrity line to leave our comfort zone and stake claim to usefulness as we should.

PHILIPPINES 3:14 I PRESS TOWARD THE MARK FOR THE PRICE OF THE HIGH CALLING OF GOD IN YESHUA THE MESSIAH.

In the event we open our eyes, ears and HEART to capture a momentary view of GOD'S vision, our lives will be vitally restored, healed and elevated in Victory to carry on HIS DIVINE MISSION. GOD'S VISION will transform our walk and talk to secure eternal life and a dynamic personality as we sojourn here. We will have an anointed, purposeful air to speak, walk and talk in boldness and unconditional love and become confident to deal wisely and understand GOD'S mission in our lives.

People of destiny can not be side tracked, perhaps sometime enticed with false promises but even though they look another way and get off track they are quick to repent and make necessary adjustments to get back on track.

In the event GOD'S vision taps our HEART we will nevermore be comfortable with anything less than fulfillment. The material things of this world will not satisfy our need and will be given little consideration. Houses, cars, properties, clothes, bank accounts can not pacify our requirement and there is nothing that will fill the void except walking in GOD'S steps. We are chartered for life and headed for victorious success for all eternity, building our treasures in Heaven.

Happiness is like a tide that flows in and out that will return to us as we throw it out to others for it is in giving that we will receive. As we pass a cup of cold water to the thirsty and extend a helping hand to the down trodden, we do also to the MASTER. In being straight forward with others we will share joys with those who smile and bear sorrows with those who cry and are down trodden. As we throw flowers at all who pass our way our own world will sparkle with a fragrance and softness like newly opened honeysuckle blossoms freshly kissed by the morning dew.

ROMANS 12:15 "REJOICE WITH THEM THAT DO REJOICE AND WEEP WITH THEM THAT WEEP" JEWISH NEW TESTAMENT

In seeking peace we realize contentment comes from within and is determined by our attitude, behavior and reactions. A resoluteness to be cheerful can only be made in the face of opposition provided we are a Child of GOD for only OUR LORD grants peace that surpasses all understanding which will stand alongside us in the valley as well as the hill top.

Our dilemma is that we clench fast to GOD in the valley and imagine we can hide from HIM when we reach the hill top, rationalizing our disposition, thinking "we have arrived" and no longer have need of HIM. Therefore we attempt to cover our intentions and justify our piety as we drift from GOD'S prescribed will to follow our selfish desires. In that instant we step out of HIS protective covering and into rebellion that begins to mock HIS great and wonderful gift of SALVATION HE gave in THE MESSIAH.

Our decision to hide behind excuses [fig leaves]are employees sent from the devil, yet even then GOD penetrates beyond the cover into the HEART to agonize over our selection that entices us unto death. When we lean toward the fig leaves we thwart our option to follow HIM WHO is able to maintain perfect peace and health absolutely free of charge. ONE WHO purchased us at great price from sin and death and gained for us a place in HIS heavenly mansion.

Why do we choose to be a prodigal child? Why not retreat to HIS magnificent abundant life? Why not pursue HIM with the whole HEART so that HE can give us a new HEART and life?

PROVERBS 17:22 A MERRY HEART DOETH GOOD AS A MEDICINE, BUT A BROKEN SPIRIT DRIETH THE BONES.

The combined psychological and physiological views equal the psychosomatic approach to man's well being, a merry HEART and medicine is dual treatment for man's ills. THE MERRY HEART DOETH GOOD LIKE A MEDICINE bears witness to the mental factor in man's health. One of the decisive conditions of bodily health is a strong integrated personality, stemming from a glad and cheerful, hardy and noble mind.

The cheerful HEART is a good preventive as well as a reliable corrective treatment which far out weighs medicine. The contented and pleasant disposition protects against disease for the mind has a powerful influence over the body. If there are non physical factors which cause disease, then there must be non physical factors to cure it.

A merry HEART is life to mankind and will extend his days when the whole man is involved in the prevention and cure of illness where sensitivity is included and appreciated.

PROVERBS 15:15 HE THAT IS OF A MERRY HEART HATH A CONTINUAL FEAST. PSALMS 43:5 WHY ART THOU CAST DOWN, O MY SOUL? AND WHY ARE THOU DISQUIETED WITHIN ME? HOPE IN GOD; FOR I SHALL YET PRAISE HIM, WHO IS THE HEALTH OF MY COUNTENANCE, AND MY GOD. ISAIAH 35:10 THEY SHALL OBTAIN JOY AND GLADNESS AND SORROW AND SIGNING SHALL FLEE AWAY. ISAIAH 35:10

GALATIANS 6:4 BUT LET EVERY MAN PROVE HIS OWN WORK, AND THEN SHALL HE HAVE REJOICING.

All of these regulations are pertinent and significant to the HEART for it is by GOD'S design that we are created for obedience and by the intentions of our HEART we either promote or pervert our honor.

WHAT ARE WE TO OTHERS

There is a vast difference between impressing someone and making an impact upon them. Impressions are easily forgotten, while impacts leave lasting results. Until we manage to meet head on with prayer the items that will challenge Heaven to arise and push back the powers of the night EPH. 5:1-16 we set in a sad state of ignore and will never experience what can be, for only GOD can overthrow the evil intended by the monarch of hell.

The Believers life should possess a distinctive pattern intended to challenge and rebuke the contemporary society but there must be forgiveness in the family of GOD, for the Christian character finds its pattern and exemplar in GOD HIMSELF, The FATHER, WHO forgives all our sin.

Oh, man, forgive thy mortal foe, Never strike him blow for blow; For all the souls on earth that live To be forgiven, must forgive. Forgive him seventy times and seven, for all the blessed souls in heaven are both forgivers and forgiven. By: Alfred, Lord Tennyson

The Church today has a need to retain its identity by the purity of its life, to put a stop to worldly input and steer clear of evil practices and pursuits; they have a responsibility to show up by a contrasting way of life the nature of the world around them and its culpability. Christian influence should have a reproving effect to the world around to be a light on top of a hill and salt to flavor in GOD'S wholesomeness.

PSALMS 100:4 ENTER HIS GATES WITH THANKSGIVING AND HIS COURTS WITH PRAISE; GIVE THANKS TO HIM AND PRAISE HIS NAME. SEEDS OF DISCOURAGEMENT WILL NOT GROW IN A THANKFUL HEART. NIV

It was in the CREATOR'S model design that we be comfortable with a determined quality of health, energy, raw brain and natural materials which HE intended for joy. We were fashioned for HIS Pleasure to pursue HIS DIVINE NATURE and in selecting HIS WILL for our lives we without a doubt fall heir to HIS design.

Wise maintenance and a cheerful disposition will protect health, prolong life, add warmth and vibrancy to our personality and will increase success, stimulate and multiply our pleasantries. These traits are easily attainable to every person and there is no healthier remedy for the HEART.

Even though there are exceptional circumstances that call for exceptional emotions, GOD'S gift to all for comprehensive living is joy as stated by Solomon;

ECCL. 3:13 AND ALSO THAT EVERY MAN SHOULD EAT AND DRINK, AND ENJOY THE GOOD OF ALL HIS LABOR, IT IS THE GIFT OF GOD.

Dr. Marshall Hall said long ago that cheerfulness was better than anything we could acquire at the drug store and he frequently prescribed just cheerfulness for his patients.

"Mirth is GOD'S Medicine and everyone ought to bathe in it" A phase once spoke by a wise man in his 90's by the name of Bancroft.

As we till the soil or plant the seed of our daily lives we will strive to see nutritious bread, not wasted toil and when clouds appear we will determine to see silver linings that will water our seed, not fear a destructive storm. Even though occasionally the whole shebang appears faulty and battered on every side we must remember that GOD does not abandon HIS own, HIS thoughtfulness is higher than ours and HE unceasingly does what is for our best.

It doesn't take a genius to understand that if we desire good health we eat healthy foods, in correct amounts. WE do not cram ourselves with junk foods, dope, nicotine, soda pop or the like or we are inviting bad health, even death. Without healthy food to nourish the body the brain can not properly perform or believe.

The same principle relates to the eye that will allure the mind and penetrates the HEART. If we desire a healthy mind and HEART we will reject looking, reading, doing or even thinking evil. We will not allow jealousy, pride and hateful things to center our thoughts, for the intent is to make the HEART sick. [steal, kill & destroy]

An elementary standard for reliable hygiene is cleanliness. While the washing of hands is not a spiritual or Biblical need it is often necessary to block the spread of bacteria and the like. Germ warfare can be avoided by washing our hands thus we resist the danger of possible foul matter or waste products that could readily be passed from the hands to the mouth or on to others that could produce infection and disease.

A popular sin of this era is sexual activities with multiple partners. Many performing erotic acts that embrace handling, tasting or even digesting refuse products from another's body such as oral sex or homosexuality, the un-natural use of GOD'S intended purpose for the body [Romans 1:18-22]. How revolting that one would place what should be the cleanest part of the body, the mouth on someone else's genitals that GOD prepared specifically as a passage to discharge waste from the body. GOD considered the waste from the body so corrupt, HE called it dung.

Today intellectual minds of wisdom have constructed vast plants to extinguish the stench and death defying germs that come from human waste [dung] yet humans kiss and manipulate those areas of the body as if cherished. Should we wonder why GOD is encompassing us with warnings in deadly disease, pestilence, earth quakes, storms, drought, etc.?

While other intellectual minds have determined to justify homosexuality under the guise of an alternate lifestyle. But it is usually the final stage in any civilizations which turns from GOD. Many feel that the act of sodomy finds its root foundation and interpretation from the City of Sodom which GOD destroyed for the unspeakable act of sodomy and that sodomites are firmly established in evil personified. GOD burned the City of Sodom off the world maps and the act is still considered an abomination by GOD.

Sodom is a charge and sentence in one word. It is a disaster site meant for all the world to acknowledge in fear. All who condone and entangle themselves with this evil exploit will provoke GOD to remove HIS divine protection and allow the adversary to shackle and blind them in a place where depravity becomes a way of life. This corrupt life style will either damn the soul for eternity or cause one to be so repulsed by the demoralized adulterated activity as to turn from it into repentance for the sake of SALVATION.

ROMANS 1:24 THIS IS WHY GOD HAS GIVEN THEM UP TO THE VILENESS OF THEIR HEARTS' LUSTS, TO THE SHAMEFUL MISUSE OF EACH OTHER'S BODIES. :25 THEY HAVE EXCHANGED THE TRUTH O GOD FOR FALSEHOOD, BY WORSHIPPING AND SERVING CREATED THINGS,

RATHER THAN THE CREATOR - PRAISED BE HE FOREVER.
JEWISH NEW TESTAMENT

The sympathy between body and soul though framed of contrasting elements are amazingly close and what effects one will hasten to the other. So when we feast on unhealthy foods or waste appropriate only for burning the affects will detail an afflicted body and diseased mind. It will affect body functions and cause reasoning to be radically disassociated from wisdom. The relationship of body and soul can not be separated as long as they are housed together as one.

We must keep a lookout on our eyes. Straying eyes lead to straying minds and are most vulnerable to temptation's attack.

In the midst of this sin-ravaged generation, a clarion call comes from Heaven to rise up, take in hand the Sword of Truth and enter the obedient fight of faith for good health and eternal life as we sojourn here that will enable us to seize victory for life by the authority granted to us by YESHUA. This is not the hour to slumber or set passively by and anticipate any outside intervention to miraculously rescue us. It is a matter of SALVATION as well as a matter of the HEART and the only way we will arise victoriously is first to kneel down in prayer.

satan WHO?

Man's attitude today toward demons is likened to his attitude in the dark ages toward bacteria.

PLAYBACK: Year   1666   Place: London

> Theme: Bubonic Plague is at it's height.
>
> Cause: People are told the culprit is fresh air.

The sight and sound of the city are like the climax of a horror movie. Palls of black smoke hang over the city as people sit in tight scaled chambers and burn foul smelling messes toward off fresh air.

Modern man has adopted similar belief today toward the demon world. They refuse to accept the fact as written in GOD'S WORD that we are in the grip of satan and his countless host of invisible demons to aid him in his dark design for man.

As Americans sit back in almost total denial of demons, TV and movies are invaded with shows to demonstrate evil almost to horrible to look at and yet people pour into movie houses or rent videos that make the promoters of hell fat, rich and able to produce more trash to poison minds of those who never heard about THE SAVIOUR.

There is hardly a culture, tribe or society to be found in this world that does not have some concept or fear of an invisible evil power. This has been attested to by Christian missionaries and secular anthropologists alike.

Witch doctors, shrunken heads, voodoo dolls, and totem poles all give dramatic evidence of this universal fear. While many today even doubt satan's existence as he is evidenced in cartoons, dolls, toys and anything that makes money while bringing satan more glory and destroying minds of countless millions.

Even Flip Wilson has made a fortune causing millions to laugh with his famous 'the devil made me do it' line.

While most see the devil as a medieval and mythical two horned, fork-tailed impish creature, dressed in red flannel underwear, he uses and taunts, haunts, and terrorizes millions who are innocently his victims or his workers of iniquity.

Believers everywhere are to be witnesses to the truth of the GOSPEL according to the prayer of YESHUA John 17. We need to be a committed community of faith which loves and serves together for the blessings of GOD are for those who share in HIS values and purpose.

The body is effected regularly by the intellect, for example a fatigued physique is usually caused by a broken spirit, a physical nausea can produce worry and the loss of appetite is normally rooted in sorrow.

Acute illness and ailments of many who are convalescent are believed to originate in the mind. Outstanding physicians have made this claim for years, just as modern science has proven that mental moods have the power to produce disease and poor health.

Today's generation is convulsed in sin. A generation of academic excellence, unmatched technical skill and unsurpassed technological development that has pushed aside and forgotten GOD WHO is the giver of all we have, even the air we breathe.

We are engulfed in immoral retrogression, secular humanism, financial upheaval and political instability and it's hard to stay above the tide if we are not disciplined to make GOD'S WORD a priority each day.

Just as food is strength to the body, GOD'S WORD is health, food and power to the spirit meant to be consumed daily. When the body and mind are not accurately nourished they will diminish and grow frail and feeble because what affects one, also effects the other.

Experiments at the University of Oklahoma, under the direction of Dr. Chesterfield G. Gunn, show that what goes on in the brain has a bearing on what goes on in the arteries and to perpetuate evil is destructive to the system but to establish a good and positive lifestyle is beneficial and profitable for producing good health and strength.

Scientific test point to the complex role of the nervous system, in accelerating arteriosclerosis and the triggering of HEART attacks. In one experiment in which two groups of rabbits were fed exactly the same low-fat diets, the scientists stimulated with electrodes a certain part of the brain of one group. This gave off tiny electrical discharges which stimulated nerve impulses. The results were very revealing, in three months the stimulated group's cholesterol had risen three times as much as the other group and the fat deposits in the arteries had accumulated four times as much. Because of their abrupt experience with the electrodes, they developed fear and coupled with pain they became anxious and afraid.

The general conclusion is that the anxious, easily-excitable, over competitive person is more prone to HEART attack than the calm person. We live today in the midst of a:

MATTHEW 17:17 YESHUA ANSWERED, PERVERTED PEOPLE, WITHOUT ANY TRUST! HOW LONG WILL I BE WITH YOU? HOW LONG MUST I PUT UP WITH YOU? BRING HIM HERE TO ME! JEWISH NEW TESTAMENT

We have become so desensitized by situations we have allowed to intrude through the constant bombardment of evil on TV, the movies as well as everyday existence that we are no longer offended or humbled to hear the most heinous of assaults occurring in our own lives. What once shocked us we now pay no mind too. As mounting violence surrounds us and crime rapidly increases these assaults forge a permanent picture in the mind that has brought us to a time when we have grown to expect them.

PROVERBS 30:14 A BREED WHOSE TEETH ARE SWORDS, WHOSE JAWS ARE KNIVES, READY TO DEVOUR THE POOR OF THE LAND, THE NEEDY AMONG MEN. JEWISH TANAKH

If we are not firmly established in GOD'S WORD a trauma can result in HEART failure as many are experiencing because the HEART is the throne of 'all' the consequences of life and what we treasure and cling to will determine happiness or gloom, faith or doubt, life or death.

The CREATOR designed each to make every moment count realistically and gave the fatiguing emotions of fear, anger, anxiety and sorrow. The fact that we were supplied with such qualities confirms that every last one is designed for a specific time to be displayed and each emotion is with in our realm of control to be used in the context of wisdom and restrained for the time appointed.

ECCLESIASTICS 3:1-8 TO EVERY THING THERE IS A SEASON, AND A TIME TO EVERY PURPOSE UNDER THE HEAVEN :2 A TIME TO BE BORN, AND A TIME TO DIE; A TIME TO PLANT, AND A TIME TO PLUCK UP THAT WHICH IS PLANTED;

:3 A TIME TO KILL, AND A TIME TO HEAL; A TIME TO BREAK DOWN, AND A TIME TO BUILD UP; :4 A TIME TO WEEP, AND A TIME TO LAUGH; A TIME TO MOURN, AND A TIME TO DANCE. :5 A TIME TO CAST AWAY STONES, AND A TIME TO GATHER STONES TOGETHER; A TIME TO EMBRACE, AND A TIME TO REFRAIN FROM EMBRACING; :6 A TIME TO GET, AND A TIME TO LOSE; A TIME TO KEEP, AND A TIME TO CAST AWAY; :7 A TIME TO TEAR, AND A TIME TO SEW; A TIME TO KEEP SILENCE, AND A TIME TO SPEAK; :8 A TIME TO LOVE AND A TIME TO HATE; A TIME OF WAR AND A TIME OF PEACE.

Anger and fear were designed for moral and ethical use but we often distort them to cause our destruction. They were intended to be used as emergency powers, to be employed for bodily protection much like the porcupine who stiffens his quills in the face of jeopardy as he hustles without hesitation away from any exposure. We usually lack the wisdom to follow the prudence of the porcupine when danger arises, we also fall short of lifting GOD'S Standard to face jeopardy or retreat as briskly as possible in the Authority GOD has bestowed upon us.

It is within our weakness and undivided faith in GOD that HE will entrust HIS angels for our safekeeping and it is by HIS wisdom that we will know what our response shall be in each event. Regardless of whether we run from or stand boldly to celebrate HIS Standards and to expose the evil that confronts us.

PSALMS 34:8 THE ANGEL OF THE LORD CAMPS AROUND THOSE WHO FEAR HIM AND RESCUES THEM. JEWISH TANAKH

PSALMS 35:5 LET THEM BE AS CHAFF IN THE WIND, THE LORD'S ANGEL DRIVING THEM ON. JEWISH TANAKH

Rather than flee the exposure of evil to many choose to grandstand in self-pride to oppose the enemy, they stand robustly face-to-face with disaster in their own strength and ignorance. The consequence of such a foolish and stubborn decision only positions us with out protection for even though GOD is our safeguard, HE calls pride an abomination and rejects any part of it, HE will not tolerate or abide by it.

PROVERBS 8:13 TO FEAR THE LORD IS TO HATE EVIL; I HATE PRIDE, ARROGANCE, THE EVIL WAY AND DUPLICITY IN SPEECH. JEWISH TANAKH

In a self-exalted state of pride the blood circulation will inflate and increase glucose, fabricated by fury and panic that will empower the muscle for use in a conflict or a challenge, the peripheral ischemia and the decrease in the blood clotting theme lessens the consequences of the wounds that may be generated in combat. But even so, we stand alone in the pride of our own vigor rather than GOD'S.

FLESHLY CONFLICT WITH GOD

The WORD of GOD frequently appears in conflict with man's hereditary and cultivated traits of character as well as his manner of life. Consequently the HEART has a rugged assignment accommodating or receiving elements and provisions for the happy HEART.

Each in our own way can acquire happiness, peace and tranquillity in our individual world whether it be good or bad because we are awarded that capability, but the only way to progress from a environment of frustration to a world of peace is inter-change within. We are incapable of obtaining peace unless we submit to GOD in HEARTFELT repentance and allow HIM to gain entry to change the HEART'S desires.

GOD deals undeviatingly with the HEART and the association will emulate as a reflector what the HEART savors and is devoted too, to wit we live richly or decay affirming the preference we make in the concealed man, the HEART. Our existence is dedicated abundantly to the inner desires of that SEAT OF PASSION.

Tranquillity and cheerfulness are personal assets as well as qualities to be sought after, therefore we should search within ourselves to encounter them. We must embrace and profess them until they mature and become second nature. But to often we camouflage them with anger, pain, selfishness, worry, bitterness and the like, creating self torment and disappointment.

If we suppose skepticism we will deteriorate and be downcast but if we adopt virtuous and confident assurance, we will prosper and be appreciative. Our foremost confidence must be saddled in GOD as our CREATOR, PROVIDER, HEALER, etc., subsequently we have no doubt in ourselves and others according to HIS WILL. We will understand that we must acquit others by virtue of the fact that we have been so greatly forgiven for there is freedom from disease for the HEART and great peace in forgiveness.

The genuine example of health or abundance is not what we invest in or attain on earth but in our approach to GOD and what we render to HIS KINGDOM. Each of us are accountable for what we think, who we are and what we have faith in. We determine what is inside our HEART by the encumbrances we consent to penetrate and adopt in our sense of right and wrong. As the old adage relates "Trash in, trash out" associates appropriately to mind and body. It is in rejection of HIS WORD that we are told

TITUS 3:9 BUT AVOID FOOLISH QUESTIONS, AND GENEALOGIES, AND CONTENTIONS, AND STRIVINGS ABOUT THE LAW; FOR THEY ARE UNPROFITABLE AND VAIN :10 A MAN THAT IS AN HERETIC AFTER THE FIRST AND SECOND ADMONITION REJECT :11 KNOWING THAT HE THAT IS SUCH IS SUBVERTED, AND SINNETH, BEING CONDEMNED OF HIMSELF. TITUS 1:16 THEY PROFESS THAT THEY KNOW GOD; BUT IN WORKS THEY DENY

HIM, BEING ABOMINABLE, AND DISOBEDIENT, AND UNTO EVERY GOOD WORK REPROBATE.

GOD gave a singly and unique mind to each one. A thought factory where our deliberations are kept inside or turned out. Our merriment or anguish holds fast to what we give credence to or discredit, whether positive or negative it is our personal 'free-and-easy' decision of choice.

PROVERBS 23:7 FOR AS HE THINKETH IN HIS HEART, SO IS HE.

Our emotions are a thermostat that permits us to warm up or cool off, to be optimistic and cheerful or pessimistic and sorrowful relative to the daily challenges of life. What we consider as true can change our entire personality and philosophy.

There is zest for life built into faith in GOD. "It is faith and enthusiasm in something that makes life worth looking at" said Oliver Wendell Holmes

There is immense benefit in happiness, peace and joy and GOD is the author of each. A healthful physique and intellect is priceless and all these attributes are embedded in the pure and wise HEART. A HEART that looks for GOD the Giver and taker of life is the wisest of all HEART'S and will enjoy life abundantly.

PSALMS 29:11 THE LORD WILL GIVE STRENGTH UNTO HIS PEOPLE; THE LORD WILL BLESS HIS PEOPLE WITH PEACE.

We can not purchase happiness, joy, peace, a sound mind, body or HEART from drugs nor any physician for only the Supreme GOD assigns them freely without cost to HIS Children. HE is a good FATHER - WHO hovers around HIS own.

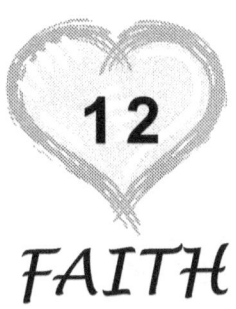

FAITH

This globe is brimming in frustration, insecurity and ill-defined lives that will find no contentment or salvation without faith. Faith will provide wings to advance above our self made anguish to sore with the eagles. Feelings of disappointment and rejection can not weigh us down for the LORD is our source and HE makes all things good.

No scattered life can be brought into focus in a maze of hesitance and compromise but if we pull ourselves together and become faithful, each step we travel toward GOD, our lives will become more secure an elevated to health, harmony and happiness.

An individual who clings to a pessimistic temperament or a disorganized personality is a casualty of cynical opinions fabricated by reservations and fright which are implements of war from satan that generates evil darts designed for our annihilation. There is but one antidote and that is allegiance with GOD it is the only unfailing panacea for anxiety, self-pity, self depreciation, inferiority, pessimism, apathy and fear.

Faith in GOD will produce assured competence and position us above the screaming affliction of this world, it will furnish us with vigorous effectiveness to dwell, walk and communicate in diplomacy.

As we submit in confidence to GOD we will be fortified, encouraged and capable of defying and dealing with evil slings and arrows aimed at us from the enemy. Even offensive utterances cast by friends, family, neighbors and strangers meant to demoralize our intellect and speeded along by the accuser will be defeated when we walk in GOD'S Wisdom as the foundation of knowledge. GOD assumes our hardship because we are HIS and HE will carry the load of trails and gloom when we allow HIM. HE will encourage and exalt us to a superior foundation far above distressing problems. HIS blessings are met within the eternal distance of repentance.

ISAIAH 53:4 YET IT WAS OUR SICKNESS THAT HE WAS BEARING, OUR SUFFERING THAT HE ENDURED. JEWISH TANAKH

ISAIAH 63:9 IN ALL THEIR TROUBLES HE WAS TROUBLED, AND THE ANGEL OF HIS PRESENCE DELIVERED THEM. IN HIS LOVE AND PITY HE HIMSELF REDEEMED THEM, RAISED THEM, AND EXALTED THEM ALL THE DAYS OF OLD :10 BUT THEY REBELLED, AND GRIEVED HIS HOLY SPIRIT; THEN HE BECAME THEIR ENEMY AND HIMSELF MADE WAR AGAINST THEM. JEWISH TANAKH

Hardships are commonplace and GOD issues enough wisdom into each HEART to know its own peril of hopelessness and the need for faith to be courageous. Just as each back knows its burdens and needs confidence to lighten the load and each eye has limited view and must maintain diligent guard of the baggage allowed to enter the mind by way of the eye. Diligent review must be made to assure correctness so that we do not promenade about deceived and permit chicanery to enter the royal seat of our HEART to rule.

The BIBLE is YESHUA, and the only LIVING BOOK that can penetrate, cleanse and conform the body to make it alert and lively and will bestow to us wisdom by discernment. "IT" makes us conscious of satan's deceit intended to trip and seduce us into hell and damnation. But when THE WORD sets on a shelf for decoration and remains unopened and unread, "IT" can have no significance for "THE LIVING WORD" is designed to be our daily spiritual food and nourish our Spirit in confidence, to keep us vigilant and supply vigor to challenge another struggle with our head prominent because we know GOD is our effectiveness and with HIM all things are possible.

JOHN 1:14 THE WORD {YESHUA} BECAME A HUMAN BEING AND LIVED WITH US AND WE SAW HIS SH'KHINAH {GOD'S MANIFEST GLORY}.

It is often said that 'seven days make one week but seven days without prayer makes one weak.'

13

CARELESS GOSPEL

With sympathy we should articulate affection and never cease forewarning those who consider a careless gospel as 'OK'. Those who are moronic enough to believe that GOD sent HIS ONLY SON to sacrifice HIMSELF for them but assume it un-necessary to seek HIS WILL by way of HIS WORD are deceived and hence hurl their destiny to the wind, for they have become wise in their own eyes as they go forth to challenge final judgment for their favored deception.

ROMANS 1:22 CLAIMING TO BE WISE, THEY HAVE BECOME FOOLS. :23 INFACT, THEY HAVE EXCHANGED THE GLORY OF THE IMMORTAL GOD FOR MERE IMAGES, LIKE A MORTAL HUMAN BEING, OR LIKE BIRDS, ANIMALS OR REPTILES. :24 THIS IS WHY GOD HAS GIVEN THEM UP TO THE VILENESS OF THEIR HEARTS' LUSTS, TO THE SHAMEFUL MISUSE OF EACH OTHER'S BODIES :25 THEY HAVE EXCHANGED THE TRUTH OF GOD FOR FALSEHOOD, BY WORSHIPPING AND SERVING CREATED THINGS,

RATHER THAN THE CREATOR, PRAISED BE HE FOREVER AMEN. JEWISH NEW TESTAMENT

In their opinion the urgency to know GOD is not a mandatory need and to attend a good BIBLE believing Church isn't in their agenda, consequently they pursue and spread their own gospel, which is accursed and condemned by YESHUA.

There is no toleration for legalism with the LORD and those who espouse the law in light of legalism are guilty of placing others into the same bondage and condemnation they carry. For they are bound by the cords of their sin and their crime against humanity. Their ultimate eternal home will be among those screaming and gnashing their teeth in the fire of hell and there will never, never be a relief.

GALATIANS 1:11 FURTHERMORE, LET ME MAKE CLEAR TO YOUR, BROTHERS, THAT THE GOOD NEWS AS I PROCLAIM IT IS NOT A HUMAN PRODUCT; :12 BECAUSE NEITHER DID I RECEIVE IT FROM SOMEONE ELSE NOR WAS I TAUGHT IT, IT CAME THROUGH A DIRECT REVELATION FROM YESHUA THE MESSIAH. JEWISH NEW TESTAMENT

GALATIONS 2:16 EVEN SO, WE HAVE COME TO REALIZE THAT A PERSON IS NOT DECLARED RIGHTEOUS BY GOD ON THE GROUND OF HIS LEGALISTIC OBSERVANCE OF TORAH COMMANDS, BUT THROUGH THE MESSIAH YESHUA'S TRUSTING FAITHFULNESS. THEREFORE, WE TOO HAVE PUT OUR TRUST IN MESSIAH YESHUA AND BECOME FAITHFUL TO HIM, IN ORDER THAT WE MIGHT BE DECLARED RIGHTEOUS ON THE GROUND OF THE MESSIAH'S TRUSTING FAITHFULNESS AND NOT ON THE GROUND OF OUR LEGALISTIC OBSERVANCE OF TORAH COMMANDS. FOR ON THE GROUND OF LEGALISTIC OBSERVANCE OF TORAH COMMANDS, "NO ONE WILL BE DECLARED RIGHTEOUS. [PSALM 143:2]" JEWISH N.T.

GALATIONS 2:21 I DO NOT REJECT GOD'S GRACIOUS GIFT; FOR IF THE WAY IN WHICH ONE ATTAINS RIGHTEOUSNESS IS THROUGH LEGALISM, THEN THE MESSIAH'S DEATH WAS POINTLESS. JEWISH NEW TESTAMENT

This message was brought to life by Paul at the risk of death, for Paul had been 'chief of sinners' when he served the Roman Government, but now he served GOD. Here he gives testimony of what GOD'S consecrated work had accomplished in his life for Paul had the Damascus road experience where The LORD had knocked him to the ground and blinded him for three days thus he knew first hand of the LORD'S power to strike down or exalt.

Not only is a sinner saved by grace through faith in YESHUA but the saved sinner lives by grace. Grace is a way to life and a way of life. GOD pardons sinners by faith and then preserves them by faith.

GALATIANS 3:11 NOW IT IS EVIDENT THAT NO ONE COMES TO BE DECLARED RIGHTEOUS BY GOD THROUGH LEGALISM, SINCE "THE PERSON WHO IS RIGHTEOUS WILL ATTAIN LIFE BY TRUSTING AND BEING FAITHFUL. [HABAKKUK 2:4]". JEWISH NEW TESTAMENT

GALATIANS 3:17 HERE IS WHAT I AM SAYING; THE LEGAL PART OF THE TORAH {TEACHING LAW, PENTATEUCH}, WHICH CAME INTO BEING 430 YEARS LATER, DOES NOT NULLIFY AN OATH SWORN BY GOD, SO AS TO ABOLISH THE PROMISE. :18 FOR IF THE INHERITANCE COMES FROM THE LEGAL PART OF THE TORAH, IT NO LONGER COMES FROM A PROMISE. BUT GOD GAVE IT TO AVRAHAM THROUGH A PROMISE. :19 SO THEN, WHY THE LEGAL PART OF THE TORAH? IT WAS ADDED IN ORDER TO CREATE TRANSGRESSIONS, UNTIL THE COMING OF THE SEED ABOUT WHOM THE PROMISE HAD BEEN MADE.

MOREOVER, IT WAS HANDED DOWN THROUGH ANGELS AND A MEDIATOR. :20 DOES THIS MEAN THAT THE LEGAL PART OF THE TORAH STANDS IN OPPOSITION TO GOD'S PROMISES? HEAVEN FORBID! FOR IF THE LEGAL PART OF THE TORAH WHICH GOD GAVE HAD HAD IN ITSELF THE POWER TO GIVE LIFE, THEN RIGHTEOUSNESS REALLY WOULD HAVE COME BY LEGALISTICALLY FOLLOWING SUCH A TORAH. :22 BUT INSTEAD, THE TANAKH {HEBREW SCRIPTURES, OLD TESTAMENT} SHUTS UP EVERYTHING UNDER SIN; SO THAT WHAT HAD BEEN PROMISED MIGHT BE GIVEN, ON THE GROUND OF YESHUA THE MESSIAH'S TRUSTING FAITHFULNESS, TO THOSE WHO CONTINUE TRUSTINGLY FAITHFUL. JEWISH NEW TESTAMENT

As YESHUA declared "IT IS DONE" on Calvary HE proclaimed HIS WORK on Earth complete, the promise of safe passage into that Holy City was established. HE WHO IS AND WAS AND IS TO COME had prepared the way and holds the key to the entrance of eternity.

YESHUA'S mission was completed as HE gave up HIS SPIRIT at Calvary {MATTHEW 15:37}. HE had paid a price HE did not owe for our SALVATION as HE captivated supreme payment within HIS BODY by HIS BLOOD for our REDEMPTION [ROMANS 3:21-26]. HE had paid a debt we can never repay and made it possible for believers to be delivered from the penalty of death, hell and the grave set forth by the Torah/Law for disobeying it. The MESSIAH redeemed us at Calvary from the curse pronounced by the Torah/Law as HE became cursed on our behalf and we have the legal right to claim our SALVATION, the sad fact is most donot even realize HIS Glory.

GALATIANS 3:13 THE MESSIAH REDEEMED US FROM THE CURSE PRONOUNCED IN THE TORAH BY BECOMING CURSED ON OUR BEHALF; FOR THE TANAKH SAYS,

EVERYONE WHO HANGS FROM A STAKE COMES UNDER A CURSE. JEWISH NEW TESTAMENT

The Torah/Law is a frame work of grace [ROMANS 6:14-15;8:2] it is man in rebellion who faults as he misuses and perverts GOD'S Law into a framework of legalism or judgment, usually in order to justify his gain, greed or lusty desires.

A healthy individual will flourish in an environment deadly to someone who is sick, likewise the Law, is beneficial to a believer who lives richly by faith but is a device of doom to one who is controlled by a sinful nature, unbelievers can not help but reject it's contents as well as IT'S MESSIAH.

A prime example of divine faith is found in Daniel Chapter 3 as the three Hebrew boys who walked in faith in the ONE TRUE GOD refused to bow to the powerful King Nebuchadrezzar who had constructed a golden statue 90 feet high and 9 foot wide of himself to cause others to honor him and his gods.

As the scheduled day of dedication for this majestic statue began, the king had obligated every VIP in the empire to assemble in the Plain of Dura to celebrate and glorify this sculpture, he had employed an orchestra to play and at the sound of music all his subjects were commanded to fall down and worship his image.

Failure to comply with the King's wishes would result in certain death by being thrown into the burning furnace. The Romans executed criminals through crucifixion, the Jews by stoning and the Babylonians by burning {Jer. 29:22} What an alter call!

The Hebrew boys Shadrach, Meshach and Abednego refused to bow and were immediately reported to the king by jealous Babylonian officials. {Daniel 3:3-8}. In answer to these allegations the young men left no doubt that they would not bow to the gods of the King nor to the King. {Daniel 3:16-18}

The boys knew they could have bowed down and found forgiveness but choose, at the risk of possible death to hold up GOD'S WILL and HIS STANDARD and told the King "Our

GOD is able". Their faith towered and GOD rewarded them as the King demanded that the fire be turned up seven times hotter than normal for the young men.

To the King's wonderment as he peered into the furnace, he saw another also in the fire. A fourth man stood among the blazing flames and yet none were in torment? How is it that these three boys and the fourth were standing peacefully among the flames and yet the soldiers who had thrown them into the furnace were burned? {Daniel 3:22-24} The King speaks in amazement:

DANIEL 3:24 THEN KING NEBUCHADNEZZAR WAS ASTONISHED AND, RISING INHASTE, ADDRESSED HIS COMPANIONS, SAYING, DID WE NOT THROW THREE MEN, BOUND, INTO THE FIRE? THEY SPOKE IN REPLY, SURELY O KING. :25 HE ANSWERED, BUT I SEE FOUR MEN WALKING ABOUT UNBOUND AND UNHARMED IN THE FIRE AND THE FOURTH LOOKS LIKE A DIVINE BEING. :26 NEBUCHADNEZZAR THEN APPROACHED THE HATCH OF THE BURNING FIERY FURNACE AND CALLED SHADRACH, MESHACH, ABEDNEGO, SERVANTS OF THE MOST HIGH GOD, COME OUT! :28 NEBUCHADNEZZAR SPOKE UP AND SAID, BLESSED BE THE GOD OF SHADRACH, MESHACH, AND ABEDNEGO WHO SENT HIS ANGEL TO SAVE HIS SERVANTS WHO, TRUSTING IN HIM, FLOUTED THE KING'S DECREE AT THE RISK OF THEIR LIVES RATHER THAN SERVE OR WORSHIP ANY GOD BUT THEIR OWN GOD. JEWISH TANAKH

As the boys came from the furnace everyone gathered around to see them whose bodies the fire had no effect on, whose hair had not been singed, whose shirts looked no different, to whom not even the odor of fire clung?

These young men walked by faith and believed, and GOD delivered them. This kind of 'faith' is seized only by those whose HEART is touched by GOD'S HOLY SPIRIT and will hasten to be obedient and seek HIM with all their HEART and become subservient to HIS WILL.

DANIEL 3: HOW GREAT ARE HIS SIGNS; HOW MIGHTY HIS WONDERS. HIS KINGDOM IS EVERLASTING AND HIS DOMINION ENDURES THROUGHOUT ALL GENERATIONS, A TRUTH THAT ALL SHOULD SEEK.

JEWISH TANAKH

GOD'S generosity of HIS legal process is a performance of grace bestowed upon us as a guide-line for a beneficial life and a lively HEART. We share a trust relationship with GOD and are concealed by HIS Grace where legalism has no position. We must resolve in our HEART to establish our wealth in Heaven by seeking HIS FACE and WILL. The faithful will delight within the framework of the Law [ROMANS 2:12 GAL. 3:23]and be in joyful subjection to 'SCRIPTURE'

GALATIANS 1:8 BUT EVEN IF WE, OR, FOR THAT MATTER, AN ANGEL FROM HEAVEN! WERE TO ANNOUNCE TO YOU SOME SO CALLED 'GOOD NEWS' [GOSPEL] CONTRARY TO THE 'GOOD NEWS'{BIBLE} WE DID ANNOUNCE TO YOU, LET HIM BE UNDER A CURSE FOREVER. JEWISH NEW TESTAMENT

Any gospel that does not identify YESHUA as the LAMB of GOD is deceptive and capable of drawing those who are not firmly established in GOD'S WORD into perdition [hell]. Those who for a time begin to travel the avenue of SALVATION but discontinue reading SCRIPTURE to seek GOD will be seized by the enemy who will anoint them with self-righteousness instead of GOD righteousness are in danger of damnation.

GOD'S WORD is absolute truth which matters absolutely. In "HIS WORD" alone is found the only completely dependable SHEPHERD that can give everlasting life. Consequently the

CHRISTIAN BIBLE will influence all who read "IT" and will draw them aside from death. Unfortunately what most perceive in the present as gospel is no more than legalism and tradition and both are based on malicious principles.

GOD will grant acceptance to all through the BLOOD of HIS SON YESHUA and reckons each as righteous and deserving to come into HIS presence through that Atoning Blood. Apart from putting our faith in GOD, relying on and accepting HIS design there is no SALVATION and no other means to enter Heaven.

GOD condemns those who endeavor to discredit or destroy HIS SCRIPTURE. Those who, in defiance of truth after mature consideration choose for any reason to sermonize a different gospel will not be spared and will gain their chastisement in the end with their father the devil. In their unwillingness to repent they have subjected themselves to a trap of the enemy whose aim is to steal, kill and destroy. {John 10:10}.

JOHN 10:9 YESHUA SAYS, I AM THE GATE; IF SOMEONE ENTERS THROUGH ME, HE WILL BE SAFE AND WILL GO IN AND OUT AND FIND PASTURE. :10 THE thief {satan} COMES ONLY IN ORDER TO STEAL, KILL AND DESTROY; I HAVE COME SO THAT THEY MAY HAVE LIFE, LIFE IN ITS FULLEST MEASURE. JEWISH NEW TESTAMENT

There is powerful dichotomy between acquiring GOD'S approval and humanistic favor and we surely must know the difference.   We can not afford to go through life as the drifter who slides in and out of GOD'S purpose as a gypsy because in the end the wandering nomad will be found in hell, not heaven.

A genuine relationship with the LORD gains a healthy spirit and a HEART of appreciation for the MASTER. One who is enthusiastic about learning and consuming HIS WORD. Being built up and surrounded by faithful ones who serve HIM and are ready and willing to go out into the harvesting alleys and byways to uplift, encourage and summons others to HIS KINGDOM in the love of YESHUA, not condemnation or judgment. For judgment will come soon enough as they go before GOD to justify their service to the LAMB. There are no perfect ones who walk this earth, the only perfect ONE that was ever here is YESHUA thus no one in this world has a right to look down upon another.

ROMANS 14:10 YOU THEN, WHY DO YOU PASS JUDGMENT ON YOUR BROTHER? OR WHY DO YOU LOOK DOWN ON YOUR BROTHER? FOR ALL OF US WILL STAND BEFORE GOD'S JUDGMENT SEAT; :11 SINCE IT IS WRITTEN IN THE TANAKH, "AS I LIVE, SAYS ADONAI {LORD}, EVERY KNEE WILL BEND BEFORE ME, AND EVERY TONGUE WILL PUBLICLY ACKNOWLEDGE GOD. {ISAIAH 45:23}" :12 SO THEN, EVERYONE OF US WILL HAVE TO GIVE AN ACCOUNT OF HIMSELF TO GOD. JEWISH NEW TESTAMENT

14

WHO IS lucifer?

Once, long ago lucifer was a powerful angelic GOD created arch-angel until he led a wicked revolt in Heaven against GOD in an insane attempt to dethrone the rightful MONARCH, the SOVEREIGN GOD. While his treachery proved unsuccessful, nevertheless it introduced into this universe a evil element.

EZEKIEL 28:11 THE WORD OF THE LORD CAME TO ME; :12 O MORTAL, IN TONE A DIRGE OVER THE KING OF tyre [hell] AND SAY TO him. THUS SAID THE LORD GOD: you WERE THE SEAL OF PERFECTION, FULL OF WISDOM AND FLAWLESS IN BEAUTY. :13 you WERE IN EDEN, THE GARDEN OF GOD; EVERY PRECIOUS STONE WAS your ADORNMENT; CARNELIAN, CHRYSOLITE, AND AMETHYST; BERYL, LAPIS LAZULI, AND JASPER; SAPPHIRE, TURQUOISE, AND EMERALD; AND GOLD BEAUTIFULLY WROUGHT FOR you, MINED FOR you, PREPARED THE DAY you WERE CREATED. :14 I CREATED you AS A CHERUB WITH OUTSTRETCHED SHIELDING WINGS; AND you RESIDED ON GOD'S HOLY MOUNTAIN; you WALKED AMONG STONE OF FIRE. :15 you

WERE BLAMELESS IN your WAYS UNTIL WRONGDOING WAS FOUND IN you. :16 BY your FAR FLUNG COMMERCE, you WERE FILLED WITH LAWLESSNESS AND you SINNED. SO I HAVE STRUCK you DOWN FROM THE MOUNTAIN OF GOD, AND I HAVE DESTROYED you, O SHIELDING CHERUB, FROM AMONG THE STONES OF FIRE. :17 you GREW HAUGHTY BECAUSE OF your BEAUTY, you DEBASED your WISDOM FOR THE SAKE OF your SPLENDOR; I HAVE CAST you TO THE GROUND, I HAVE MADE you AN OBJECT FOR KINGS TO STARE AT. :18 BY THE GREATNESS OF your GUILT, THROUGH THE DISHONESTY OF your TRADING, you DESECRATED your SANCTUARIES. SO I MADE A FIRE ISSUE FROM you, AND IT HAS DEVOURED you; I HAVE REDUCED you TO ASHES ON THE GROUND, IN THE SIGHT OF ALL WHO BEHOLD you. :19 ALL WHO KNEW you AMONG THE PEOPLES ARE APPALLED AT YOUR DOOM. you HAVE BECOME A HORROR AND HAVE CEASED TO BE FOREVER.

JEWISH TANAKH

GOD had created lucifer {satan} as "the anointed cherub that covereth" and GOD had appointed him a guardian cherub, as one of three arch-angels meant to operate under YESHUA as Heaven's Prophet but lucifer rose up in pride, in his HEART he became power-crazed and he transgressed against the LORD his GOD.

In coveting GOD'S strength and power satan enlisted a third of Heaven's angels and fought for his own will, however he did not desire the feeding and leading attributes for good that GOD'S Will testifies of. But we can not take lightly that GOD conquered the devil in Heaven because THE LORD also gave satan opportunity to rule the world for a period of time and today satan is known as the 'god of this world'

Even so, the strength of satan is powerless to challenge YESHUA because of his defeat at Calvary. A Child of GOD has total victory over the enemy satan and it is built into repentance and knowledge of GOD'S WORD to proclaim and hold tight to the SALVATION by faith and obedience.

The fate of satan is in the Hands of GOD and when we are Children of GOD we walk in divine protection and revelation to proclaim victory over our Father's Enemy.

ISAIAH 14:12 HOW ARE you FALLEN FROM HEAVEN, O SHINING ONE, SON OF DAWN. HOW ARE you FELLED TO EARTH, O VANQUISHER OF NATIONS. :13 ONCE you THOUGHT IN your HEART, i WILL CLIMB TO THE SKY; HIGHER THAN THE STARS OF GOD i WILL SET my THRONE. i WILL SET IN THE MOUNT OF ASSEMBLY, ON THE SUMMIT OF SAPHON; :14 i WILL MOUNT THE BACK OF A CLOUD, i WILL MATCH THE MOST HIGH. :15 INSTEAD, you ARE BROUGHT DOWN TO SHEOL, TO THE BOTTOM OF THE PIT. JEWISH TANAKH

LUKE 10:18 YESHUA SAID TO THEM, I SAW satan FALL LIKE LIGHTENING FROM HEAVEN.

JEWISH NEW TESTAMENT

It was lucifer, the prince of darkness who first became deceived and carelessly thought to occupy GOD'S Throne. In his haughty egoism, arrogance, conceit, self-love and importance lucifer elevated and regarded himself as superior to GOD.

For his absurdity he was thrust from the highest Heaven and perhaps instantly GOD prepared an inferno known as hell and lucifer became it's monarch. It is a region blazing with a fire whose hunger for the soul of man is never satisfied, prepared for satan and his followers or any who prides themselves in their own importance, being superficial about THE LORD'S GOSPEL. Hell is a domicile shrieked with pain and fiery flames where any who follows or chooses to practice evil will spend eternity with no hope.

Pride is one of satan's many tools of manipulation and it is specified as an abomination to GOD. It is a poison stitch sent into our intellect by the monarch of hell for the purpose of destruction that always causes those who fall pry to its lure needless pain and misery. It can cost us all we hold precious when we refuse to submit and surrender to the LORD. We can be confident that satan understands pride and how it effects those who parade in it. For satan also knows THE WORD in greater depth than we and he uses it on us and through us to deflate one another through legalism or criticism, etc. For he is the ancient impostor and the father of lies from the creation of time and more than proficient with SCRIPTURES that we are not even conscious of, but even 'he' trembles in the light of GOD'S WORD.

JAMES 2:19 YOU BELIEVE THAT "GOD IS ONE? . JEWISH NEW TESTAMENT

DEUTERONOMY 6:4   GOOD FOR YOU! THE DEMONS BELIEVE IT TOO, THE THOUGHT MAKES THEM SHUDDER WITH FEAR! JEWISH TANAKH

We too should tremble that ONE so Unique and Supreme as GOD would love us so much that HE could forfeit HIS ONLY SON for our eternal SALVATION. Should HE also tolerate our taking for granted such a gift as to mock it, a symbol of HIS LOVE so precious and eternal?

The proof of the pudding is still in the eating. The only test of a man's salvation is through his works. A silent believer may be indeed considered a saint before GOD, but he remains a sinner before man until he walks the walk and talks the talk of Christian service.

"Unproductive faith cannot save, because it is not genuine faith. Faith and works are like a two-coupon ticket to heaven. The coupon of works is not good for passage, and the coupon of faith is not valid if detached from works." {source: Ryrie Study Bible. P. 421}

A FOOL IN A FIX??

The rich farmer mentioned in James 12:16-21 was called a fool by GOD for he thought he could satisfy his eternal soul with materialistic goods but the only real soul food is the WORD of GOD. The farmer had misplaced his confidence in his worldly goods and thus had set his HEART upon them.

LUKE 12:34 FOR WHERE YOUR WEALTH IS, THERE YOUR HEART WILL BE ALSO. JEWISH NEW TESTAMENT

How sad for the fool who sets up his morality and responsibility in himself, for this fool GOD will make it apparent how bankrupt possessions can be. It is the one who seeks GOD with the whole HEART, the GOD-fearer who truly appreciates GOD'S position and power that has the confidence to face opposition as to make it laughably pathetic, for it is faith in GOD'S SPIRIT that is alive in the HEART that makes the difference. If we only have knowledge of HIM in our intellect it is equivalent to being with out SALVATION as long as we will not allow HIM to enter the HEART.

REVELATION 3:20 BEHOLD, I STAND AT THE DOOR, AND KNOCK; IF ANY MAN HEAR MY VOICE AND OPEN THE DOOR, I WILL COME IN TO HIM, AND WILL SUP WITH HIM AND HE WITH ME. :21 TO HIM THAT OVERCOMETH WILL I GRANT TO SIT WITH ME IN MY THRONE, EVEN AS I ALSO OVERCAME, AND AM SET DOWN WITH MY FATHER IN HIS THRONE. KJV

To pursue GOD'S Kingdom is to set a goal in life on GOD HIMSELF and the execution of HIS purpose to convey HIS standard with all its blessings, for GOD promises to fulfill the longings of such persons, and HE does not lie. Our HEART disposition will resolve our rank in life on Earth as well as our permanent destiny.

Only GOD can once and for all stop the HEART to take the life of a man. Whether he be a GODLY man or one who anticipates retirement in luxury and is content to set back engrossed in his wisdom to stroke his back for the bumper harvest "he" has harvested. As he lies back in satisfaction and conceit master minding a larger barn for storage he will unexpectedly observe that GOD is in authority and that GOD alone grants or over powers according to mans HEART posture.

JEREMIAH 17:5 THUS SAID THE LORD: CURSED IS HE WHO TRUSTS IN MAN WHO MAKES MERE FLESH HIS STRENGTH AND TURNS HIS THOUGHTS FROM THE LORD. JEWISH TANAKH

JEREMIAH 17:7 BLESSED IS HE WHO TRUSTS IN THE LORD, WHOSE TRUST IS THE LORD ALONE. JEWISH TANAKH

The wealthy man trusted his flesh and failed to gain the riches of a equitable relationship with GOD. In his insolvency he rendered himself a buffoon, a godless and ridiculous man whose HEART had solidified and became callous and condemned by reason of self-regard. The HEART that is frozen is hardened and will not allow the flow of Blood for life, nor will "IT" be able to comprehend the blessings SCRIPTURE will yield to those who embrace GOD'S instructions.

LUKE 21:26   AS PEOPLE FAINT WITH FEAR AT THE PROSPECT OF WHAT IS OVERTAKING THE WORLD; FOR THE POWERS IN HEAVEN WILL BE SHAKEN. :27 AN THEN THEY WILL SEE THE SON OF MAN COMING IN A CLOUD WITH TREMENDOUS POWER AND GLORY   :28 WHEN THESE THINGS START TO HAPPEN, STAND UP AND HOLD YOUR HEADS HIGH; BECAUSE YOU ARE ABOUT TO BE LIBERATED.   JEWISH NEW TESTAMENT

LUKE 21:26   MEN'S HEARTS FAILING THEM FOR FEAR, AND FOR LOOKING AFTER THOSE THINGS WHICH ARE COMING ON THE EARTH; FOR THE POWERS OF HEAVEN SHALL BE SHAKEN. KJV

The most essential commodity today is not speculation or despair but readiness for the end of the world as we interpret it. Life or death will be GOD'S contribution to accommodate what the HEART has arrayed itself with in the conclusive journey of eternity. As the disasters, famine and the like become common place in the world they usher in the end of time as we know it, nevertheless Believers can be filled with hope in contrast to the fear which will characterize the unbeliever.

LUKE 6:45 THE GOOD PERSON PRODUCES GOOD THINGS FROM THE STORE OF GOOD IN HIS HEART, WHILE THE EVIL PERSON PRODUCES EVIL THINGS FROM THE STORE OF EVIL IN HIS HEART. FOR HIS MOUTH SPEAKS WHAT OVERFLOWS FROM THE HEART.   JEWISH NEW TESTAMENT

Moral behavior comes out of the treasure of a virtuous HEART. It is as absurd to expect worthy fruit from a diseased tree as it is to require good conduct from a corrupt man. Only the man whose HEART is sufficiently prepared by obedience can convey good instruction. HEARTS which are committed in obedience to GOD through HIS SON YESHUA will journey into Heaven where there will be celebrated ecstasy and divine sanction, no more affliction, grieve, depression, anguish, corruption or dying. A City where the roadways are gold and the light will be as jasper, clear as crystal. [REV. 21:11; 4:3;3:18]

GUARANTEED ACCURACY

GOD IS the ALPHA and the OMEGA, the beginning and the end. HIS CHARACTER guarantees the accuracy of this revelation and the assurance of the consummation it heralds. The generous covenant added reverberates back a conclusive promise to the believer who remains faithful. For only the confirmed and sincere will be granted the journal entry of the Holy City in the millennium, the new creation will be his inheritance.

ISAIAH 55:1 COME ALL WHO ARE THIRSTY, COME FOR WATER, EVEN IF YOU HAVE NO MONEY; COME, BUY FOOD AND EAT; BUY FOOD WITHOUT MONEY, WINE AND MILK WITHOUT COST. JEWISH TANAKH

Those who find themselves in selection of another gospel will pass into perdition. They are the cowardly who revere man and reject YESHUA. Their reverence to the antichrist is linked to the faithless, renegade and pagans, the polluted and abominable and their final destiny will be the never-ending pit of hell-fire for the worship of idols, which is the option of their HEART.

No one actually desires death particularly if they are destined for an eternity of torture but GOD will not put up with any person that floats about in his own hypocrisy, that vagabond will accompany satan into the lake of fire.

There is no secondary alternative manner for atonement. Only damnation awaits the unbeliever and the terrifying prospect of judgment is the object of that divine wrath and it will be displayed against all who oppose GOD.

According to the Old Covenant anyone who outfits themselves in rebellion [idolatry] will suffer the penalty of death without mercy. We can not predict an altered approach to sin for an apostate. Anyone who deliberately renounces and opposes the truth of GOD'S WORD given in testimony and authored for our model will endure a much worse penalty for having rejected THE SON OF GOD. For HE gave HIS LIFE as an offering for our transgression and left a written Manuscript forged by HIS BLOOD in 'THE WORD' which HE WAS.

JOHN 1:14 THE WORD BECAME A HUMAN BEING AND LIVED WITH US, AND WE SAW HIS SH'KHINAH, {GOD'S MANIFEST GLORY} THE SH'KHINAH OF THE FATHER'S ONLY SON, FULL OF GRACE AND TRUTH. :18 NO ONE HAS EVER SEEN GOD; BUT THE ONLY AND UNIQUE SON, WHO IS IDENTICAL WITH GOD AND IS AT THE FATHER'S SIDE, HE HAS MADE HIM KNOWN. JEWISH NEW TESTAMENT

The persistent sinner who deliberately and willfully mocks GOD repudiates the sacred significance of the BLOOD which is the Covenant Seal of our sanctification. In his denial he treats the SPIRIT of GOD with prideful insolence, WHO is HIMSELF the Author of grace. Even as lucifer raised himself up in loftiness while he held the position of arch angel, thinking himself to be above GOD, so too does the unbeliever when he espouses illusions to justify the embrace of his own choice instead of GOD'S WILL.

GOD'S CHARACTER will administer judgment and show by HIS perception who are HIS people and who are traitors and rebels and for those who hold fast to HIM in trust by faith He will grant permanent perfection in Heaven. A place prepared for a prepared people with faithful HEARTS who not only proclaim GOD through HIS SON YESHUA but labor in relation to the HOLY SPIRIT of peace, love and health with out skepticism.

SIN UNCONFESSED IS SIN UNFORGIVEN

There is nothing as important as the preparation of our soul from the HEART. It is the HEART that grips the issues of life that we must safeguard from the exposure and rudiments of a sinister world management and design.

MARK 8:36 FOR WHAT SHALL IT PROFIT A MAN, IF HE SHALL GAIN THE WHOLE WORLD BUT FORFEITS HIS LIFE? JEWISH NEW TESTAMENT

To the Pharisee, Scribes, Sadducees and the self-righteous this represented a hard saying, a choice of gaining the riches of this world for a short term or being alive for all eternity in total perfection? Heaven designates total self-denial which means the complete dethronement of self so that our life will be centered around YESHUA. Surrender and submission is the surest and most abiding gain.

GOD prepared {1} an Instructor {2} a Sacrifice for sin and {3} a High Priest in HIS ONLY SON YESHUA and labeled HIM 'HIS WORD'. The MASTER OF THE UNIVERSE had sanctioned the iniquity of all and placed it on the back of HIS ONLY SON WHO gave HIS LIFE unto death at Calvary and in compassion sent back HIS HOLY SPIRIT as a guide for all who would submit to walk by faith in HIM. This reality was documented by inspired and devout men so that each of us could be encouraged to examine and inhabit it.

After the death of YESHUA the disciples eventually came to see that the cross, which had represented such a stumbling block to them, was in fact the only door available whereby eternal life was gained. It was the sign and secret of the conquest over the HEARTS of men, and thus of the coming of the kingdom.

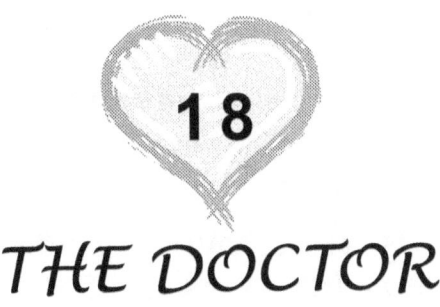

THE DOCTOR

New Testament LUKE was a doctor of medicine but unlike most practitioners his objective was to proclaim YESHUA'S humanity. Luke, a Gentile became a Jewish Proselyte converted by Paul and was known as the beloved physician. He is thought to have been a man of affluence who traveled with Paul. {Phil. 24}

Luke's qualifications for his notable ministry were manifold but above and beyond all else, he had the inspiration of the Holy Spirit. His medical training had taught him to be accurate and he was known as the faithful recorder, reliable, historian, scholarly, skillful and sympathetic. He was the recorder of the books of Luke and Acts and gives prominence to the sympathy and socialableness of YESHUA as the Man who came to rescue in Luke 15:1 and 19:10. He presented YESHUA as the true Representative of universal man.

LUKE 19:10 FOR THE SON OF MAN CAME TO SEEK AND SAVE WHAT WAS LOST. JEWISH NEW TESTAMENT

The features of Luke's gospel are clearly defined in Luke 1:28 and LUKE 2:40 as the gospel of pardon and redemption given freely in the highest degree. YESHUA is before us as the Healer of shattered HEARTS and the Sharer of woes in great sympathy. In Luke 1:14; 2:10,13; 15:7 there is great joy as Luke praises GOD while Angelic joy rings prominent as the Church vocalizes songs of thanksgiving and high praise taught to them by Luke. In his Gospel [Luke] we also find reference to special missions of the SPIRIT.

Luke's aspirations unceasingly give glory to YESHUA in every area of life and in Luke 5:31 & 32 where he recorded a vital message for doctors as well as the world.

LUKE 5:31,32 IT WAS YESHUA WHO ANSWERED THEM; "THE ONES WHO NEED A DOCTOR AREN'T THE HEALTHY BUT THE SICK. I HAVE NOT COME TO CALL THE RIGHTEOUS, BUT RATHER TO CALL SINNERS TO TURN TO GOD FROM THEIR SIN." JEWISH NEW TESTAMENT

All things are subservient to the Authority of YESHUA. When the above statement was spoken in Luke 5 YESHUA was withdrawing from the Synagogue where HE had healed Simian's mother-in-law and many others. HE silenced the cries of the demoniacs because HE wanted people to learn for themselves who HE was. In the mornings HE could scarcely escape the crowds, but nevertheless left them. The assignment for which HE had been sent by GOD to declare was the good news of GOD'S rule far and wide and HE could not linger in one region to become the idol of an admiring throng.

The WORD of GOD teaches that fear, anguish, depression and the like are by-products of evil and synonymous with transgressions. Just as a stone is thrown into a tranquil serene lagoon and begins to ripple waves in a ring-shaped fashion, slowly encircling toward the bank in all directions thus does sin as it ripples from the point of origination, outwardly to involve and often destroy all that is in its path.

The cultivation of sin initiates in the HEART encircling it with a crystallization process that continues from within to all who are near thus inducing hardness of the HEART and arteries that will eventually close out the life blood. Wrong thinking and doing is the rock thrown into the HEART that effects the life. It is contagious, poisonous and deadly as it envelopes the life in an effort initiated by the accuser for our ultimate destruction.

A wicked individual obsessed by an evil spirit today would undoubtedly be regarded as suffering from mental illness. This however, is not a full diagnosis of the phenomena in the Gospels where the demoniacs also possessed a supernatural knowledge of things unknown to the ordinary man. The presence of an evil, supernatural power can not be rationalized away and just as theologians speak of the 'concursive' action of the HOLY SPIRIT in men, so we may perhaps argue for a like action by evil spirits.

In LUKE 5:34 The HOLY ONE of GOD means the same as the SON of GOD and there are many lessons of YESHUA'S healing power in the NEW TESTAMENT, such as:

LUKE 8:41 THEN THERE CAME A MAN NAMED YA'IR {JAIRUS} WHO WAS PRESIDENT OF THE SYNAGOGUE. FALLING AT YESHUA'S FEET, HE PLEADED WITH HIM TO COME TO HIS HOUSE:42 FOR HE HAD AN ONLY DAUGHTER, ABOUT TWELVE YEARS OLD; AND SHE WAS DYING. :49 A MAN CAME FROM THE PRESIDENT'S HOME TO TELL HIM HIS DAUGHTER WAS DEAD. :50 YESHUA SAID, "DON'T BE AFRAID, GO ON TRUSTING AND SHE WILL BE MADE WELL. :54 BUT HE TOOK HER BY THE HAND, CALLED OUT, LITTLE GIRL, GET UP AND HER SPIRIT RETURNED. JEWISH NEW TESTAMENT

and again in:

LUKE 9:42 EVEN AS THE BOY WAS COMING, THE DEMON DASHED HIM TO THE GROUND AND THREW HIM INTO A FIT. BUT YESHUA REBUKED THE UNCLEAN SPIRIT, HEALED THE BOY AND GAVE HIM BACK TO HIS FATHER. :43 ALL WERE STRUCK WITH AMAZEMENT AT THE GREATNESS OF GOD. JEWISH NEW TESTAMENT

YESHUA stresses the opposition to evil, perhaps as the bearer of the HOLY SPIRIT. For YESHUA is the SHEPHERD WHO knows HIS SHEEP. HE leads, saves, satisfies, died for and today unites HIS SHEEP. Such a sacrificial commitment by a SHEPHERD is in stark contrast to the hireling, whose only real interest is personal gain. Hired hands may watch over the sheep when it is to their advantage, but they will not risk their life to protect someone else's property .

19

DIVINE HEALING

Today a high body temperature is referred to as a technical medical term and has cost unbelieving millions of dollars to regulate while The ALMIGHTY GOD looks down in wonderment and grief, speaking regularly through HIS WORD "LOOK TO ME, LET ME GIVE YOU NEW LIFE, A NEW HEART. COME OUT OF DARKNESS FOR YOUR HEALING, I SENT MY SON FOR YOUR SIN, INIQUITIES AND INFIRMITIES, BY HIS STRIPS YOU WERE HEALED" HE is the Almighty Healer yet ignored, YESHUA lives today healing the diseased and delivering the lost.

In MARK 1:30 we find high body temperature to be a evil spirit thrust upon mankind by the enemy, yet subjected to YESHUA'S authority again in

MARK 1:30 SHIM'ON'S MOTHER-IN-LAW WAS LYING SICK WITH A FEVER, AND THEY TOLD YESHUA ABOUT HER. :31 HE CAME, TOOK HER BY THE HAND AND LIFTED HER ONTO HER FEET. THE FEVER LEFT HER, AND SHE BEGAN HELPING THEM. JEWISH NEW TESTAMENT

When we know YESHUA and submit to HIS WILL with the whole HEART, HE will heal and deliver us from sinful enslavement, provide security, preserve us and convert our HEART'S condition and craving. As we draw nearer to HIM WHO is our SALVATION we will recognize the Authority given through HIS sacrifice at Calvary to articulate in HIS NAME and defy the prince of darkness. So that satan and his immoral infantry will evacuate our life and remove all his depraved behavior, affliction, plagues and the like.

HEBREWS 10:12 BUT THIS ONE, YESHUA, AFTER HE HAD OFFERED FOR ALL-TIME A SINGLE SACRIFICE FOR SIN, SAT DOWN AT THE RIGHT HAND OF GOD. 13 FROM THAN ON TO WAIT UNTIL HIS ENEMIES BE MADE A FOOTSTOOL FOR HIS FEET 14 FOR BY A SINGLE OFFERING HE HAS BROUGHT TO THE GOAL FOR ALL TIME THOSE WHO ARE BEING SET APART FOR GOD AND MADE HOLY. JEWISH NEW TESTAMENT

By the simple act of repentance we are adopted into the household of GOD, YESHUA'S HEAVENLY FATHER becomes our HEAVENLY FATHER. We are prepared by the unblemished, hallowed, righteous BLOOD of YESHUA [as the sacrifice for our sin] to go in the presence of A HEAVENLY FATHER, seek HIS FACE and request in faith for HIS PROVISIONS.

The passage to GOD'S Royal seat was opened at the death of YESHUA as HIS FLESH was lacerated. How GOD'S HEART must have ruptured to observe the pain and suffering of HIS ONLY SON sinking towards death with all the transgression of the world laid upon HIS Back. In GOD'S grief HE ushered HIS distaste of HIS own creation as:

LUKE 23:44 DARKNESS COVERED THE WHOLE LAND UNTIL 3 IN THE AFTERNOON :45 THE SUN DID NOT SHINE ALSO THE PAROKHET [CURTAIN] IN THE TEMPLE WAS SPLIT DOWN THE MIDDLE. CRYING OUT WITH A

LOUD VOICE YESHUA SAID "FATHER! INTO YOUR HANDS I COMMIT MY SPIRIT". JEWISH NEW TESTAMENT

YESHUA'S fate was a planned and unique action for SALVATION. The period was of HIS choosing as HE delivered HIS SPIRIT into the HANDS of HIS FATHER so that even Pilot marveled that HE expired so quickly. MK 15:44 and JOHN 10:11.

When the veil[curtain] was rent[torn] GOD opened the HOLY OF HOLIES to all of mankind that would acknowledge and enter by way of HIS SON WHO is the Sacrifice that paid our sin debt.

HEBREWS 10:19 SO BROTHERS WE HAVE CONFIDENCE TO USE THE WAY INTO THE HOLIEST PLACE OPENED BY THE BLOOD OF YESHUA :20 HE INAUGURATED IT FOR US AS A NEW AND LIVING WAY THROUGH THE PAROKHET [CURTAIN] BY MEANS OF HIS FLESH :21 WE ALSO HAVE A GREAT COHEN [HIGH PRIEST] OVER GOD'S HOUSEHOLD :22 THEREFORE LET US APPROACH THE HOLIEST PLACE WITH A SINCERE HEART IN THE FULL ASSURANCE THAT COMES FROM TRUSTING [FAITH] WITH OUR HEARTS SPRINKLED CLEAN FROM A BAD CONSCIENCE AND OUR BODIES WASHED WITH PURE WATER. JEWISH NEW TESTAMENT

Marks Gospel 27:51-53 has recorded the split of the Temple curtain, signifying right of entry into the presence of GOD. This accomplished labor of love performed by YESHUA is also recorded in Matthew's version. YESHUA arose from death as the FIRST FRUITS , the graves of others opened and they too, rose up from their graves.

Free access to GOD'S presence was manifest as the temple veil was torn. SALVATION was fixed and became accessible to mankind when YESHUA died at Calvary. HE had crushed the enemies bondage and bestowed HIS authority upon HIS followers for the defeat of satan and as HE was seated at the right hand of HIS FATHER, HE took HIS rightful place as our High Priest and

Advocate. Through HIM we are deemed righteous and deserving to petition The LORD.

YESHUA TOOK HIS PLACE AT HIS FATHER'S SIDE TO BECOME OUR HIGH PRIEST. AND THE POSITION OF THE EARTHLY PRIEST WAS PUT AWAY COL. 1:20-22.

The fact is that YESHUA "IS" the Resurrection and HE still heals the diseased and raises the dead. The faith of our HEART determines what HE is to us and what HE is allowed to accomplish in our life.YESHUA'S ability to defend and purify us and satisfy our need establishes the sincerity of purpose [a true HEART] and absolute confidence [full assurance of faith] of what HE did as it symbolizes the old ritual forms of sprinkled blood and freshly washed bodies

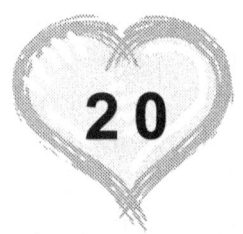

DOCTORS FOR TODAY

Doctors of medicine have a symbolic capacity to improvement this world and those who recognize this task are the physicians that are worthy of much applause as long as their work harmonizes with GOD'S.

The competent practitioner can administer aid for healing by setting a broken bone, sewing a torn body, removing a cancerous lump in the system, change the appearance, perform a heart transplant, open veins for blood to flow unhindered with the benefit of tools and perform many other necessary aids for recovery but they are powerless to render healing, for that comes from the one and only Divine Healer, YESHUA THE MESSIAH [JESUS CHRIST].

Conscientious physicians do their foremost to be about healing but it is GOD who cleanses or allows one to pass on into eternity. For the saint, no one knows the reasons they are called home to Heaven. Perhaps they have completed their project here on earth, satisfied their season and traveled on to their reward. Or perhaps even through they are saved, they decline to perform so GOD takes them out of harms way? For the unbelievers, the devil's order and purpose is death as he strives to steal, kill and destroy GOD'S SEED from infancy.

There is no denial that doctors are a necessity and there are assuredly circumstances that GOD has programmed for their charge, nevertheless for to long villainous men of medicine have denied recovery to many due to covetous intents of profit. Physicians can deceive their patients in many ways by misrepresenting the facts as he sees them or withholding data. Such deceptions are morally unlawful and are considered theft because they keep the patient from the rightful truth.

They have rejected GOD'S delivering and recovering omnipotence from dread of either not knowing HIM or not wanting to know HIM. That is a conscience conclusion granted to each of us, to seek or deny HIM.

In most cases if it were not for the weak, much of the profession of medical science would not flourish and many physicians would be unable to afford the fineries of life such as elegant cars, country club living, exclusive clothing and luxuries. The lust of the flesh, lust of the eyes, the pride of life could not be fulfilled with out liberal fees, thus the immoral doctors minister healing at a minimal significance to imprison a profitable sufferer for return visits to pad their pocketbooks.

Doctors who patronize the abomination of abortion and the euthanasia of the elderly are guilty of the execution of the most inoffensive and faultless of society. They have regressed into a league of greedy, nauseating and repulsive life form, but those who refuse to stand up and speak out, who set by quietly watching this detestable practice are also condemned by their apathy and will answer at Judgment for their passive insensitive indifference.

1 SAMUEL 15:23 FOR REBELLION IS LIKE THE SIN OF DIVINATION {WITCHCRAFT}, DEFIANCE, LIKE THE INIQUITY OF TERAPHIM. BECAUSE YOU REJECTED THE

LORD'S COMMAND, HE HAS REJECTED YOU.
JEWISH TANAKH

The refusal to acknowledge this travesty of murder performed on the innocent and elderly by professional peers screams in a deafing silence to be heard. Those who prevail in utter stillness, feeling they are detacted from this lampoon find themselves couched in guilt by association. They have placed their hands into evil by their refusal to grandstand and articulate 'against' such unspeakable acts. Their stubbornness and unwillingness to speak up denies the standards of YESHUA and consequently their unmitigated calm is thunderous.

Instead of recognizing the evil from the summit of the good, they recognize the good from the abyss of evil and in fear shrink from exposing and condemning this disaster that has allowed AMERICA to be cursed as the blood of infants run into the streets and scream for justice. Just as Abel's blood rose from the cursed ground up into Heaven:

GENESIS 4:10 THEN GOD SAID, "WHAT HAVE YOU DONE? HARK, YOUR BROTHER'S BLOOD CRIES OUT TO ME FROM THE GROUND. :11 THEREFORE,YOU SHALL BE MORE CURSED THAN THE GROUND, WHICH OPENED ITS MOUTH TO RECEIVE YOUR BROTHER'S BLOOD FROM YOUR HAND. JEWISH TANAKH

As the Children made in GOD'S IMAGE are murdered in the name of convenience or sacrifice or greed it is their Blood that cries out for justice from the Supreme Maker and Giver of all Life. The voice of the martyred blood invokes vengeance of GOD'S Covenant and reveals the serpent's seed in our Society.

The physicians who are against this mockery, yet hang their head in shame and silence either do not realize or choose to ignore that this matter is set in the HEART of GOD WHO holds the reins to all HEARTS. And that in their unwillingness to acknowledge and speak out against these monstrous exploits of holocaust in this Nation, they condone and share responsibility for the abominable blasphemies that reign down the curses upon our Country.

It does not matter for what purpose the doctor patches or sews or transplants, GOD secures and heals and HE, WHO searches the HEART and assembles each individual in HIS Image intended each life to experience purpose. But sadly today many doctors trifle with fire as they mimic GOD in their decisions to kill or with-hold life saving facts for the sake of lining their own pocket.

PROVERBS 24:10-12 IF YOU SHOWED YOURSELF SLACK IN TIME OF TROUBLE, WANTING IN POWER. IF YOU REFRAINED FROM RESCUING THOSE TAKEN OFF TO DEATH, THOSE CONDEMNED TO SLAUGHTER; IF YOU SAY, "WE KNEW NOTHING OF IT", SURELY HE WHO FATHOMS HEARTS WILL DISCERN {THE TRUTH}, HE WHO WATCHES OVER YOUR LIFE WILL KNOW IT, AND HE WILL PAY EACH MAN AS HE DESERVES. JEWISH TANAKH

GOD will give Divine protection in exchange for up holding HIS STANDARDS of TRUTH. For those who seek HIS WISDOM will see HIS blessings and realize victory in their lives. But HE consigns to hell those who are nerveless and refuse to position and exclaim truth.

The honorable physician does recognize with certainty that their educated and accomplished labor to the flesh is not the sum total or absolute fountain of healing. They understand that the HEART of every SOUL is weighted in GOD'S HAND and that HE is the HEALER and doesn't need the doctor but the physician must have GOD'S healing balm in every case for success.

"THE CONCEPT OF HEALTH AS A NARROW PROFESSIONAL CONCERN IS OBSOLETE". DR. HULDA REGEHR CLARK, Ph.D., N.D.

By faith in YESHUA SALVATION is gained. Anything short of THE MESSIAH is deception, substandard, unfulfilling and unacceptable. No scant hypothesis of integrity or vow of discipleship will liberate a soul and we have no freedom with or right to claim YESHUA unless we are totally HIS. Feebleness in direction is derived from half HEARTEDNESS in the believers life and will give occasion to suffering. This condition arises when effort is made to promote self first and give YESHUA the left overs of life, if we deny HIM before the world, HE will deny us before HIS FATHER and no one will endure when the test comes upon him with out YESHUA

Many causes are streamlined today, ranging from religion to politics but the only solution is THE CREATOR for all issues of life come from the HEART and are under GOD'S Authority. HE is the LORD of Abundant life WHO GIVES dynamic meaning to existence. Knowing HIM and walking according to HIS will gives rise to health, it is divinely distributed and complete for there is no diverse form with GOD.

GOD does not sin, HE can not lie and HE will not change.

THE BELIEVING PHYSICIAN

There is great blessing in a Christian Doctor who believes with all his HEART that he is an assistant to the work of YESHUA. He discerns that only GOD the Creator has the authority to cure bodies, give new HEARTS, ETC.

The Christian Physician is given an awesome ministry united in discretion and integrity to nurture assignments that most of us would not ponder and they are to be admired and honored. Even so they still do <u>not</u> have the ability to produce blood, divinely eliminate a lump, insert new veins, give a new HEART, BODY, MIND. Only the MASTER CREATOR can and does work miracles for those who acknowledge HIM.

A GODLY Doctor professes and acknowledges the mastery of GOD and is found praying with and for his patients, he is one of this planets most excellent and admirable blessings and when we locate such a person, a man of GOD who is a scholarly and prudent physician, we should be compelled to pray for him as he is assuredly thrashed by the ungodly spirits of the god of this world as he collides with flesh and spirit in his plight to repair the body and lead the way to life and soul saving SALVATION for his patients.

On the contrary the unbelieving doctor is a hazard of adversity to civilization for he depends upon his own self-learned intelligence, independent of GOD the CREATOR to perform deeds on bodies created by GOD, in GOD'S own image. How does he justify doing GOD'S work of healing without GOD?

PROVERBS 9:10 THE BEGINNING OF WISDOM IS THE FEAR OF THE LORD. AND KNOWLEDGE OF THE HOLY ONE IS UNDERSTANDING.

JEWISH TANAKH

The true value of life is realized in the knowledge and service to GOD as wisdom's free and gracious invitation is set before us. The consequences of our conduct, good or bad, chiefly reflect ourselves. Those who seek wisdom will be exalted to higher ground but those who act in utter ignorance of right will sink into perdition under a millstone of guilt without remedy.

Numerous doctor's make a conscience choice to ignore GOD'S wisdom and have set a monetary value on the techniques of doctoral supervision that has given life and death a flavor of sadistic destruction. Frequently they surmise the conclusion and num us with massive doses of pain killer that dissolves our resistance against medication until all of a sudden we are in an distinguishable need for pain killer and our immune system is saturated by pain killers and a prescription for pain can not work.

It seems that moral principles have been all but abandoned by most medical professionals and bound for a dead-end, ignoring right and wrong to occupy an almost faddish place in the sun.

The context of theology can not be arranged through biology, and rewards are created by living within the guidelines of GODLY spiritual standards that far exceed man's knowledge, and are more valuable than life maintained at the cost of man's wit, corruption or depersonalization.

Innumerable pastors, doctors and professionals of today in their pursuit to become more synchronized with 'nature' and accomplished with more intellect [the enlightened mind] have chosen to ignore GOD'S WILL and in the frame of that choice they elevate themselves by their own 'illuminated wisdom' and it has created a vacuum [a trap] for the sincere minded apprentice to stumble into. More simply put, thinking themselves wise the intellectuals have become fools.

ROMANS 1:22 CLAIMING TO BE WISE, THEY HAVE BECOME FOOLS. JEWISH NEW TESTAMENT

GOOD DOCTORS WHO PRACTICE MEDICINE WITHOUT GOD

In some instances doctors who are enthusiastic and sincere of HEART do promote recovery to their foremost ability and experience. But the expression 'practicing medicine' is still all they can afford to hallo their profession for they offer no guarantees and unless they know the Divine HEALER from their HEART, all they can do is 'practice' for they have no faith and can not understand there is a Supreme HEALER. By their rejection of YESHUA they are sightless and subservient to the evil god of this world who also has great creative power.

2 CORINTHIANS 4:4 THEY DO NOT COME TO TRUST BECAUSE THE god OF THIS 'OLAM HAZEH {WORLD} HAS BLINDED THEIR MINDS, IN ORDER TO PREVENT THEM FROM SEEING THE LIGHT SHINING FROM THE GOOD

NEWS ABOUT THE GLORY OF THE MESSIAH, WHO IS THE IMAGE OF GOD. JEWISH NEW TESTAMENT

YESHUA THE HEALER

YESHUA is the Doctor who cures disease, forgives sin, wraps us in RIGHTEOUSNESS, cleanses iniquity {sin} and infirmities {sickness} and re-creates us white as snow {THE NEW BIRTH- WE ARE BORN AGAIN}. HE opens the mansion door to Heaven where perfect health is ours for eternity and even though HE was supreme, in HIS HUMAN form He could no more than a doctor be expected to keep HIS hands clean as HE walked on Earth.

LUKE 11:39 HOWEVER, THE LORD [YESHUA] SAID TO HIM "NOW THEN, YOU P'RUSHIM [PHARISEES] YOU CLEAN THE OUTSIDE OF THE CUP AND PLATE; BUT INSIDE, YOU ARE FULL OF ROBBERY AND WICKEDNESS. :40 FOOLS! DIDN'T THE ONE WHO MADE THE OUTSIDE MAKE THE INSIDE TOO?" JEWISH NEW TESTAMENT

YESHUA often made social visits to the dwellings of the Pharisees where clean hands were not associated with hygiene but believed to eliminate corrupt defilement. So concerned with tiny details of doctrine the Pharisees gave no consideration to moral principals. They were hypocrites who treasured the respect of men and elevated themselves above others with evil aspiration of self exaltation seeking their own magnificence.

Hypocrites are damned for obscuring GOD'S revelation to keep men from GOD'S Kingdom. These impostors solicit the philosophy of culture and it is a philosophy without divine revelation, at it's best it is inadequate but at its worst it is destructive to the BIBLE, human dignity and value. All Spiritual and moral truth is established in YESHUA and any other understanding is without light.

A blunder hidden in the basis of a system of thought does not become honest simply by being in full operation. It remains an inaccuracy; and if intuition is agreeable, that consistency can mean only a more twisted seduction of error as in the case of the Hypocrites.

Error requires a mistake in logic to produce correct conclusions from false premises, but counterfeit conclusions can be drawn from deceitful material with rational accuracy. In this way, entire detailed systems of opinions can be unbound in which the code of scientific procedure is quickly obeyed, and yet the whole strategy can be undermine by a delusion at its foundation.

Unfortunately there are believers who refuse to read the WORD of GOD or subject themselves to the study of it and in their withdrawal to seek, pursue and understand GOD'S WORD they are doubtlessly influenced and dazzled by the intellect and scholarship of philosophers as well as false prophets, who are obliged by their father the monarch of hell and predestined to demolish the religion of carnal believers.

Nevertheless the foundation of GOD'S WORD is firmly established in historical facts and it is GOD'S revelation to man, promises to humanity that SCRIPTURE can not and will not change.

The tax collector was religiously polluted because they manipulated others for the Romans, they were hated because they fleeced their fellowmen to line their own pockets with blatant prosperity. Much like the IRS, many preachers and politicians of today, the collectors used their public elected or appointed offices to pursue self serving gain but they were not outside the reach of YESHUA. Just as Saul{Paul} was overtaken by GOD as he traveled the highway to Damascus when GOD struck him down to his knees and blinded him. GOD ask, "Paul why do you persecute ME?" Paul knew in his HEART by that blinding experience that GOD was real. Suddenly Paul understood GOD'S power, that HE was the MASTER OF THE UNIVERSE, the MOST HIGH CREATOR with the power to destroy or make every moment count. Paul expeditiously sought the call of his HEART to become one of GOD'S most saintly followers who was unashamed to praise GOD no matter where he was. Paul never missed an opportunity to tell others of the ALMIGHTY GOD even though it would cost him his life.

We are all transgressors of GOD'S Law, not only the prostitutes, criminals, murders, but the ne'er-do-wells, self righteous, prideful, arrogant, etc. But YESHUA has authority over all and can change the HEART if we, the sinner will trust HIM. There are none unreachable or untouchable by GOD prior to death when GOD seizes the breath of life.

HEBREWS 9:27,28 JUST AS HUMAN BEINGS HAVE TO DIE ONCE, BUT AFTER THIS COMES JUDGMENT; SO ALSO THE MESSIAH, HAVING BEEN OFFERED ONCE TO BEAR THE SIN OF MANY. WILL APPEAR A SECOND TIME, NOT TO DEAL WITH SIN, BUT TO DELIVER THOSE WHO ARE EAGERLY WAITING FOR HIM. JEWISH NEW TESTAMENT

Rebellion and stubbornness are rewarded in satan's domain. The rich man who denied Lazarus cries for help during his life time, today screams for water from the pit of fire. After the death of the rich man he was found begging mercy for his loved ones who were following ungodly leaders, he was sorry that he had denied Lazarus but his grief came to late. Today he suffers as many others suffer for their rebellion and rejection they perpetrated while they lived. Their stubbornness caused them to miss the wondrous eternal life offered by YESHUA.

LUKE 16:24 HE CALLED OUT, FATHER AVRAHAM {ABRAHAM} TAKE PITY ON ME, AND SEND EL'AZAR {LAZARUS} JUST TO DIP THE TIP OF HIS FINGER IN WATER TO COOL MY TONGUE, BECAUSE I'M IN AGONY IN THIS FIRE! JEWISH NEW TESTAMENT

The rich man was disinherited and sentenced to hell because his faith was in riches and rebellious works. The population of hell is in a bottomless firey pit and have the ability to glance up into the splendor of Heaven where they will never have the privilege to enter. Sadly they will be tortured for their unkind deeds and evil acts committed to others for all eternity. Their memories will linger, haunt and torment them forever as the inferno radiates a blistering furnace in remembrance of their past behavior.

The inhabitants will roust about in the blazing pit of fire as they look into Heaven to envision the impeccable mansion they too could have had. While those in Heaven are incapable of seeing past perfection and will have no past memory of what once was.

Heaven is comfort, Hell is torment. Heaven is joy, Hell is anguish and sorrow. The servant of YESHUA will be comforted but the stubborn rebellious sinner will be tormented. Both situations are fixed in eternity and are set before us as an option prior to our final breathe.

SALVATION GAINED

GOD'S truth fulfills man's greatest practical necessity, the conversion of the soul [the HEART] through faith. But HIS inclusive principals should not to be thought too pure and holy to be brought into daily life. They are the truths which reach to Heaven and compass eternity, yet their vital influence is to be woven into everyday human experience. They should permeate all the great and small things of life.

The leaven of truth when received into the HEART will regulate the desire, purify the thought and sweeten the disposition. It quickens the faculties of the mind and the energies of the soul and enlarges the capacity for feeling and loving.

According to SCRIPTURE the principle of faith embedded and cultivated in the HEART as a way of life is pleasing to GOD and as we express, confess and persist in it the perseverance in our HEART will take full possession of its reward.   F a i t h in GOD'S sight is the one essential condition of value and it deals with two essential things of the future which are 'HOPED FOR' and 'NOT YET SEEN'. Without such an attitude of awareness and assurance towards GOD 'IT IS IMPOSSIBLE TO PLEASE HIM' to 'DRAW NEAR TO HIM' or to have personal dealings with HIM.

GOD is the supreme reality which deals with faith. HIS promises and the reward of those who seek HIM are the fulfillment of that faith.

Our HEARTS must be convinced that what GOD has inspired to be written in HIS WORD is solemn truth and only truth will make us free from the bondage of satan and his corrupt powers and the only escape from the prince of darkness is through GOD and our faithfulness to HIM.

OLD TESTAMENT HERO'S OF FAITH

Many have passed into eternity before our birth who were approved by GOD as worthy to be recorded in scripture and acted strictly by faith before YESHUA'S time. They left written testimonies in HIS WORD to serve as an example to us that GOD will protect HIS WORD from the enemy as it continues to encourage and illustrate HIS WILL. The SCRIPTURES document and are a witness that has outlived the individuals who gave their lives. Through the record of their performance their faith has spoken to others in their death.

The genuine rewards, crowns and treasures are beyond this life-span and are faith's witnesses that the dividends lie beyond death in a better resurrection. The martyrs are those who endured great suffering, who died painful and shameful deaths rather than deny their faith.

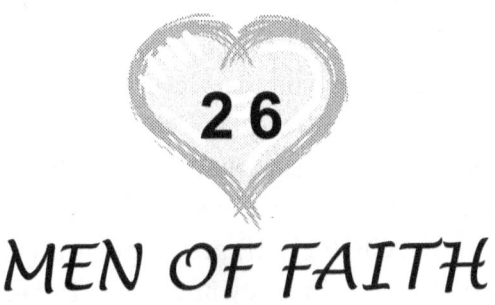

MEN OF FAITH

ENOCH = Whose faith was a witness that in this life when man's HEART so pleases GOD, HE gives an escape from death and a fuller enjoyment of HIS own presence and glory.

NOAH = A peculiarly significant example for those privileged to hear the gospel for out of reverence for a WORD from GOD which spoke of impending judgment and indicated a way of salvation, acted in obedience to the divine command because he believed that what GOD said would be fulfilled in building the ARK, Noah was counted faithful.

ABRAHAM = Obeyed the divine call to go forth to possess an inheritance, though he did not know to what land he was going, still less what it was like.

SARAH = Who was long past barren to even consider bearing a child trusted in GOD'S WORD of promise and HIS active faithfulness in fulfilling HIS WORD to give she and Abraham the promised Child.

MOSES = His parents acted in faith by placing him in a basket and setting the basket afloat in the river. GOD's provision for

Moses was met by the King's own daughter who drew the basket from the river and raised Moses as her own, when the King demanded all infant boys be put to death.

GOD'S blueprint for Moses was not thwarted as satan had planned but fulfilled as seen in SCRIPTURE when Moses grew up and led the Hebrew Nation out of Egypt through the RED SEA. All this was according to faith in GOD and recorded in the Old and New Testaments as well as the extraordinary faith chapter known as HEBREWS 11.

Mans achievement of faith is victory over satan's authority, affliction and demise but only for those willing to put away tradition, pride, stubbornness, rebellion and the like to submit to GOD in repentance unashamed to give HIM praise and GLORY.

The martyr's of SCRIPTURE are in position to give strength and intelligence of GOD'S mercy and love. Those who were unashamed to be seen glorifying the supreme GOD. These men ignored the tradition of ancestors and chose to walk with The ALMIGHTY, they refused to allow flesh and blood to chain them or others in bondage through culture and self-importance.

Our dilemma originates when we reject the reflection of HIS SCRIPTURE where HIS WILL, MERCY, JUSTICE AND DELIVERANCE are found activated according to HIS truth. In the effort to approach GOD void of the YESHUA'S Blood Covering we can not please HIM because we are clothed in filthy rags and defy HIS WILL. YESHUA'S BLOOD is the CLOAK, the only covering whereby we are found deserving and HE died to provide that Cloak for each of us.

JAMES 1:21 RID YOURSELF OF ALL VULGARITY AND OBVIOUS EVIL, AND RECEIVE MEEKLY THE WORD IMPLANTED IN YOU THAT CAN SAVE YOUR LIVES. DON'T DECEIVE YOURSELVES BY ONLY HEARING WHAT THE WORD SAYS, BUT DO IT. JEWISH NEW TESTAMENT

YESHUA can't deviate from the objects of HIS care. HE was uniquely predetermined with the power to remove filthy garments and replace them with the robe of repentance, HIS robe of righteousness. As we accept HIM - HE writes pardon against our names on the records of Heaven. He confesses us as HIS before the Heavenly universe and the monarch of hell becomes our adversary, our prosecuting attorney and the impostor that begins the comprehensive seduction. But GOD is in control and we are shadowed in HIS DIVINE PROTECTION.

LEPROSY THE RESULT OF SIN?

Leprosy can mean any of several skin diseases and is a well known symbol of sin. It is nauseatingly communicable, and spreads with frightful swiftness, its corrupting character begins with a seemingly inoffensive blemish. Its incurability so far as the wisdom of man is concerned are all witness to the inability of mans wisdom to cure.

In Lev. 13 & 14 Moses, in response to GOD'S command placed his hand in his bosom and when he with drew it, the hand was covered with leprosy. GOD repeated the instruction to Moses to place his hand again in his bosom and upon with drawing, it was clean. No sign of leprosy. This gesture was intended to instruct Moses and designed to teach Moses the extraordinary authority of his LORD; that he should be captivated, instantly with leprosy confined in his hand, and cured immediately without the use of means was an astounding wonder. It also demonstrates the perfect ease with which GOD can unexpectedly inflict a disease and just as quickly cure it and how simple a matter it was and is for ALMIGHTY GOD to ransom HIS people out of the hand of the Egyptians.

Moses' hand symbolized leprosy, it was a sign of how it can affect corrupt flesh that is under GOD'S curse.

JOEL 2:13 REND YOUR HEARTS RATHER THAN YOUR GARMENTS AND TURN BACK TO THE LORD YOUR GOD. FOR HE IS GRACIOUS AND COMPASSIONATE, SLOW TO ANGER, ABOUNDING IN KINDNESS AND RENOUNCING PUNISHMENT. MESSIANIC JEWISH TANAKH

The hand speaks of energy and is considered the instrument for work. Moses was GOD'S instrument for work. He was GOD'S resource for a phenomenal plan to bring HIS people out of Egypt. But this demonstration of the LORD was to show Moses how simple it is for GOD to set aside the flesh of mankind. It was confirmation that the energy of the natural man is not the mainspring of action in GOD'S Service.

By nature our hand is unfit to be used by THE SUPREME BEING but GOD in HIS Divine grace interposes cleansing power and that which is weak and powerless is overcome with supernatural strength; under GOD any task that is accomplished by the hand of man is manifest because of the LORD'S power.

Mankind of today are no different from the Egyptians or the Jew of Moses time, for we too are defiled and need cleansing and that purification comes through YESHUA the MESSIAH WHO is HIMSELF HOLINESS.

HE HAD NO SIN {HEBREW 4:15}, HE DID NO SIN {1 PETER 2:22} HE KNEW NO SIN {2 CORINTHIANS 5:21}

In boundless grace HE took our responsibility for sin, placed it on HIS BACK and HE became the Sacrificial LAMB to purchase for each of us eternal life. Just as the Lambs of the Old Testament carried the sin of the people into the wilderness, relieving them of the curse of sin for a season, YESHUA'S unselfish act put away our sin for all of eternity, if we will only accept and seek HIM.

EXAMPLE: Suppose you went to the hospital. Your body is filled with filthy cancerous blood cells, knowing you didn't have long to live, expecting to die soon due to your condition. Then I came in to your hospital room free of any disease. My body in excellent condition. My morals beyond reproach and my HEART in superior shape. And in my love for you and having compassion for your condition I told the doctor to with draw all of my blood and place it into your veins so that you could live and replace my blood with your blood. I would die for taking your blood into my body.

But that is what YESHUA did for each of us. HE took our cancerous sin driven flesh upon HIMSELF to the cross and left it in hell, but to acquire what HE left for us we have to submit to HIS WILL for HIS enriching and abundant life.

HE WAS MADE SIN FOR US 2 COR. 5:21

HE BARE OUR SINS IN HIS OWN BODY ON THE TREE. 1 PETER 2:24

HE DESTROYED THE WORKS OF THE devil[satan]. 1 JOHN 3:8

HE TAKES AWAY OUR SIN. 1 JOHN 3:5 JEWISH NEW TESTAMENT

We who are justified are ushered into a state of grace which brings security and confidence. A blessed by product of SALVATION is joy, a triumph based on hope and victory over affliction. We can boast in trial and tribulation because we realize our sojourn here is temporary and will eventually lead way to victory as we pass into eternal life.

A relationship with the MESSIAH is not just a feeling but a reality obtaining access to GOD'S Throne, for none are able to enter into favor with the FATHER GOD on our own merit. The presentation before GOD'S Royal Throne is effected by ONE near the Monarch HIMSELF, WHO is seated at HIS Right Hand and has opened up the way for us to go before the throne of HIS FATHER. GOD is our FATHER by adoption in Grace.

Just as we understand that suffering produces patience and endurance leads to a tested character, the proved experience ushers in hope.

ROMANS 2:7 TO THOSE WHO SEEK GLORY, HONOR AND IMMORTALITY BY PERSEVERANCE IN DOING GOOD, HE WILL PAY BACK ETERNAL LIFE.   JEWISH NEW TESTAMENT

2 TIMOTHY 2:3 ACCEPT YOUR SHARE IN SUFFERING DISGRACE AS A GOOD SOLDIER OF THE MESSIAH YESHUA. JEWISH NEW TESTAMENT

Our HEART as a believer will be flooded with love and as we study and seek GOD we will become more conscience of HIS wondrous Love toward us through the indwelling of HIS SPIRIT that will be projected to all around us. We will act different, feel changed, have more confidence and will walk on higher ground.

Anyone who rejects the Affirmation of GOD'S WORD has elected to position them self under the jurisdiction of the prince of darkness and becomes depraved by nature. In mans refusal of YESHUA he forfeits GOD'S blessings and lays hold to doom, confident of nothing but Divine Judgment as he anticipates the second and eternal death. For only the Lake of Fire awaits all who reject YESHUA.

For that purpose all who call on HIS ALMIGHTY NAME and profess to be 'Believers" should commence to petition GOD for the SALVATION of those we love. Forewarn them about the everlasting inferno that lust after their soul and the Great PHYSICIAN WHO died to deliver and ransom them from a bed of anguish or affliction? HE preferred to give HIS life.

There is no antidote for self righteousness except GOD'S righteousness. No physician has the capability of dealing with the HEART without surgical instruments, only the HOLY SPIRIT can make such a godlike achievement within us to give us the new HEART, devout life and avant-garde beginning. When GOD'S love flows in the veins, the system purifies itself and the HEART becomes new.

Still there are many who walk in vanity and haughtiness who pride themselves on excellence to credit and place their trust in the big "I", having deceived themselves of their importance. But self-righteousness is not true righteousness and all who cleave to self-exhalation will be left to the consequences of a fatal deception and those who vow to observe the Commandments of GOD but neglect the love of GOD in their HEART to others act in self righteousness.

YESHUA beckons us to join in HIS achievements for the redeeming of humanity while multitudes are comfortable with status quo doctrine as they mutter 'HINENI' {Hebrew = here am I LORD send me} yet pursue idleness. Like the unfaithful son we fabricate deceitful promises that defile our soul. We profess by declaration to be sons of GOD but in life and integrity we contradict that relationship when we fail to surrender "our will" to GOD, thus we contentedly live a lie.

A lesson to remember is that satan utilizes the listless, sleepy habitual idleness of professed Believers to strengthen his forces and influence human beings to his camp. While many think that though we do no actual work for YESHUA we are yet on HIS Side, in reality we are enabling the enemy to pre occupy ground and gain advantages. By our neglect to be diligent workers for our MASTER we leave duties undone and words unspoken and allow satan to gain control of souls who might have been won for SALVATION. Even a doctor by mending a hurt or stopping a pain can not impose SALVATION on to another, that is a HEART moved motion worked through the inspiration of the HOLY SPIRIT. But we are called to tell those around us about HIS undying love and mercy and if we are willing, HE will reward us.

Victor Hugo said, "Short as life is, we make it still shorter by the careless waste of time." We are time killers and in the end, it kills us. The sleeper who lies for hours in bed is a do-nothing and has no regard for time. He is not just lazy in work, but lazy with life in general.

GOD is the benefactor of life and HE sent HIS ONLY SON YESHUA to purchase the master key to death or new birth, our choice. But GOD is not obligated to anyone and has measured out a specific gift of time to each for service to HIM. GOD gave time wings to soar through life with an aim to perform HIS Will as an Eagle or submit to the serpent and be fated for hell and exist crippled, maimed and diseased until death only to be destined for hell after dying.

JAMES 4:14 WHAT IS YOUR LIFE? YOU ARE A MIST THAT APPEARS FOR A LITTLE WHILE AND THEN VANISHES. JEWISH NEW TESTAMENT

Time past can not be recovered, once it is gone, it is gone forever and for that reason we must learn to invest the time we have in beneficial projects that will build mansions in Heaven with thoughtful planning. Time should never be treated like money that we can't wait to spend.

Yet so much time is wasted pouting over the past. We must learn to correct wrongs from yesterday or we have accomplished nothing, not even intelligence. The law of sowing and reaping is spiritual and it dominates mankind. It makes a difference in how we live and the rules we live by.

GAL. 6:7 DO NOT BE DECEIVED; GOD CANNOT BE MOCKED. A MAN REAPS WHAT HE SOWS.   JEWISH NEW TESTAMENT

This law may be among the most important slices of advice we ever get. We can make it a fantastic promise and receive the dividends of a GOD honoring life or make it hell on earth depending upon how we decide to reap.

HOSEA 8:7 THEY SOW THE WIND AND REAP THE WHIRLWIND.

It always escorts justice and when we seek GOD in our youth and do not dribble away our dear moments of adolescence, our tomorrow's will be victorious and triumphal. We will make time count before it runs out. But if we choose to 'DO OUR THING' in selfish arrogance the gloomy fruit of our wasted years are seasoned for nothing but harvesting crops of misfortune, tragedy and affliction in our tomorrow's.

A newspaper once carried an add in the lost-and-found section that read, "Lost yesterday, somewhere between sunrise and sunset, two golden hours, each set with sixty diamond minutes. No reward, they are gone forever."

Paul tells us in:

PHILLIPPIANS 3:13-14 FORGETTING WHAT IS BEHIND AND STRAINING TOWARD WHAT IS AHEAD, I PRESS ON TOWARD THE GOAL TO WIN THE PRIZE FOR WHICH GOD HAS CALLED ME HEAVENWARD IN CHRIST JESUS THE MESSIAH.   JEWISH NEW TESTAMENT

28

WHY WERE WE CREATED?

Our creation was meant for fellowship with our SUPREME MASTER for HIS pleasure. However as beneficiary of Adam's sin we are each born into a revolution between GOD and satan, the mind[the intellect] and flesh verses the HEART.

ISAIAH 43:7 [NEVI'IM] ALL WHO ARE LINKED TO MY NAME, WHOM I HAVE CREATED, FORMED, AND MADE FOR MY GLORY. JEWISH TANAKH

The mind and flesh are satans playhouse of molestation where he baits a soul by fascination, seducing the spontaneity of the eye, the passion of the flesh and the self-importance of life as glorious fun, thus urging the HEART to connect with the festivity.

This evil spirit, the prince of darkness realizes he can mislead the HEART if we are not forged in and devoted to the LIVING WORD, YESHUA. The HEART is sanctioned for GOD and is that element of our person that harbors our soul with which the ALMIGHTY GOD reckons. Because of WHO GOD is, HE can not look up on evil or suffer any part of it, and the mutiny created by the battle within gives rise to pride as the neck[flesh] begins to stiffen in defiance and the HEART becomes hardened in an effort to protect itself in challenge to the evilness of the flesh. Even so the arrogant personality slowly gives way to conceit as it progresses into a mundane superficial personage on the road to failure brought on by the foul spirit.

As the misguided attitude advances, the HEART'S grievance weighs heavier and the perpetual aspect of defeat becomes oppressive, a fashion unintended by the Creator and rejected by the HEART [conscious]. In the act of rebellion the flesh battles for harmony with the HEART and induces this VITAL ORGAN to build a wall of protection for itself but as the struggle continues within it delivers dis-ease and friction.

By day it is a war zone but nighttime brings assault frequented by monstrous fantasies that eventually gives rise to anguish, horror, anger and bitterness to induce worry, pain, regret, etc. The continual battle within brings illness and disease.

WOE! Our mind has reached a destination of what we regard as the point of no return. Once again we have been spoofed by the adversary as we think we can no longer handle what is going on in our body and consequently in our carnal state of mind we hasten to a practicing non-believing doctor [in most cases] who guesses at the problem as he 'practices medicine' but has no actual idea that the root enigma, is sin.

Contention has preceded honorable health and guiltless reasoning to create cancer, ulcers or some awful disease that is to impenetrable for us to endure and yet it all stemmed from the battle between the flesh and the HEART concealed in the subterranean corners of the consciousness. That smallest emotion from the past which assembled the beginning dis-ease is now beyond recollection and has reorganized itself faraway from the grasp and can not to be unearthed by the eye of flesh. The satanic intruder has seated itself within our personage and is positioned for the crucial blow that will seize our fragile existence to cast our soul into the abyss.

Only the eye of GOD foresees the arch-enemy of annihilation and only a devout physician who pursues GOD'S teachings and has an understanding of the diabolical invader can understand that he is under GOD'S Authority. This doctor is receptive of GOD'S WORD in mans life and will bring to our attention the right choices as well as the reasons for our condition that have caused the failure of our health. He is wise, expedient and unafraid to explain the crisis we have brought upon ourselves by the inferior choices we have submitted to in seeking our excessive self-indulgence.

Thousands of the insightful and prudent men and numerous scholars have divested their consciousness upon the Doctrine of YESHUA and confirmed believers are under obligation to those who elect to convince us to follow GOD'S WORD, even if the end result is disagreement. The Scripture never exterminates civility and virtuous manners, instead 'it' directs us to bestow tribute to them to whom tuibute is due.

Luke was such a person, a doctor of medicine whose faith as a physician was not upon what he could do to mend a body but trust in the promise of the Divine HEALER, YESHUA.

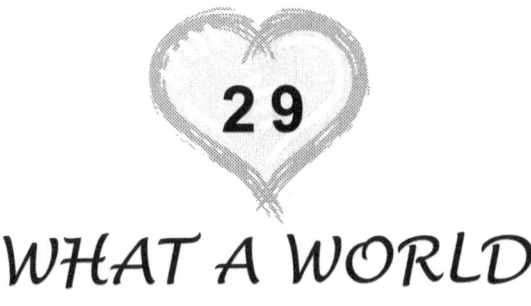

WHAT A WORLD

A great deal of man's wisdom in the present has dumped the world into a downward spiral fashioning a separation from GOD through a science oriented facet. A region where morals and medicine have become a case of average social values [problem solving] tied to cultural discipline and are a matter of economics, political science and sociology that are considered 'politically correct'.

Another viewpoint of our civilization is 'the en-lightened mind' of the professors of intellect who possess no medical credentials but wish to led society into behavioral science based on 'no god' or 'the god within' because the populace appears to be on a crusade for an explanation to the dilemmas of existence, seeking more light on ethical concepts such as motive, freedom, will, intention, determinism and value selection.

Still another perspective that assuredly warrants reference is the disgraceful allusion of the counterfeit gods of other civilizations, other cultures that have set up idolatry on American soil to the likes that we have never experienced. They have slithered their systems in to establish ground in our schools and are being taught to our children to our embarrassment.

Weakened by the adversary within and having no knowledge of GOD, many parents have abandoned the children by failing to train them in the home about the mortality of life on earth and the exemption from death available in a relationship with a GOD, WHO has even now conquered the attacker of the HEART.

PRAY FOR AMERICA

Oh where are the men of yesterday
who were not ashamed to kneel and to pray?

The women were great in virtue and modesty
they bore children with respect, Oh the yester-years of chastity....

Today's leaders push programs to stop air pollution
While morals decay, still unheeded the solution.

Prayers have been ruled out by high courts of our Land
Men of wisdom, I wonder? Do they understand?

While education of sex is taught to the babies
As pornography reins to drive us all crazy.

Cheap news is reported with lies and deceit
While acts of nobility they forget or delete.

A baby is murdered for the same of a sin
Yet most will go out and do it again.

Oh where are the men who will rise up to meet
This tide of immorality and lay it at Jesus feet?

We must see the truth in its great sensation
Our strength will be found in the goodness of our nation.

While most confirmed believers lay back embracing luxury, the cults have come into America and taken over our streets, churches, children, institutions and etc., with their depraved baggage. They have built luxurious temples trimmed in silver and gold to honor their false gods and moved onto our streets to befriend the lonely and down trodden who seek to fill a vacant place in their HEART. Consequently the idol worshipers shout and glorify their false gods as the 'church' sets back in a comfort zone full of pride and self gratification only to warm the pew each Sunday morning.

All the while we are moving further from GOD and forging distances that we can not measure much less cross until finally there is no longer even a narrow notion in our mind of the GOD WHO created us. We have become blinded by our own sin and are held by its cords.

PROVERBS 5:22 THE WICKED MAN WILL BE TRAPPED IN HIS INIQUITIES, HE WILL BE CAUGHT UP IN THE ROPES OF HIS SIN 23. HE WILL DIE FOR LACK OF DISCIPLINE, INFATUATED BY HIS GREAT FOLLY. JEWISH TANAKH

It is sobering and we are fortunate if we learn from our mistakes but in the event we pursue folly it will remove the starch out of moralism and conventional wisdom as we know it. It will drain us of our salt, our usefullness for GOD until we are no longer fit to season a world gone mad.

As unique discoveries of science come to forefront we view material systems of knowledge to detect that the training in humanities has not made us skillful enough to grasp the physics and chemistry of nuclear break through and today with the constant threat of nuclear warfare and the nuclear bomb floating from nation to nation we tremble in the apprehension of annihilation by another country.

Alerted to technology's credits and debits and the impact of that area of study, we are brought to bear the scales of value judgment and choice to confront a divided   nation that has forgotten GOD'S power and justice.

For many, medical science has become a god that controls and manipulates birth, health and death. Society has approached a juncture of no getting back to normal and in astonishment we stop to wonder, should we evade the uniform questions each day presented or invite the hazards that man's mind will continue to futurize with new experiments and methods that disallow and forbid GOD's healing measures?

Where is GOD in human wisdom but observing in bereavement as humanity giddies about, stacking one enlightened concept upon another to fashion his own tall structure of Baal that will soon tumble by confusion and abandon man leaving him expressionless and saturated with himself, without GOD. Without the ALMIGHTY, man has fabricated his own dilemma in life and death because any controversy of right and wrong, good and evil in medical care or everyday life will take us into examination relating to Christian faith.

GOD has provided each of us a personality with unique merit and HIS designs are for supreme good. HIS WILL is to be the chief medium of our knowledge of good. Life, health and death are in GOD'S HANDS yet in the 20th century many physicians have rejected medical ethics and the belief of a living GOD - WHO is the great physician. It seems that mankind has forgotten that all matters of birth, life and death are established in the Divine revelation of the Old and New Testament.

All discomfort and disease that torments us today are of divine origin - {1}to serve as an example for GOD'S Glory {2} a sin of the ancestors past down through generations or {3} a punishment, hex or even a curse.

While the root cause of our problems are divine and determined by decisions we make in life, medical studies and practice have began to assert a scientific independence of GOD and out of anxiety humans have transfer their confidence to the doctor for cure instead of GOD the SUPREME HEALER.

Where once there was a marriage of medicine and religion, today they, like most of the world stand divorced as society jumps from one marriage bed to another so too does the medical practice. Seeking remedy in many beds instead of the common bed of faith, dealing in idolatry and adultery while the only antidote is righteousness from the SEAT OF PASSION and the permanent surrender of the HEART to GOD who is MESSIAH and the CREATOR of new HEARTS, new lives, new beginnings.

Giles Ferman, a physician in the Massachusetts Colony in 1650 said, "I am strongly set upon to study divinity, my studies else must be lost; for physic is but a mean help."

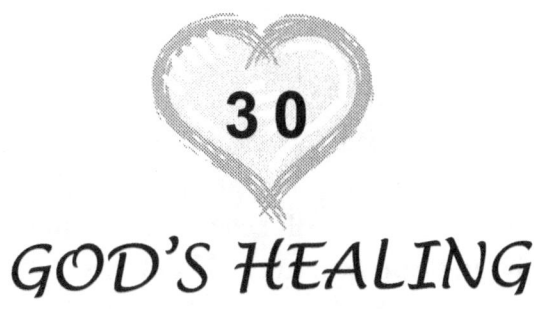

GOD'S HEALING

MAL. 4:2 THE SON OF RIGHTEOUSNESS HAS HEALING IN HIS WINGS .

Having faith in YESHUA means more than the forgiveness of sin; it means HIS taking away sin and filling the vacuum with the grace of HIS HOLY SPIRIT. It issues Divine illumination in the rejoicing of GOD. It is a HEART emptied of self and blessed with the abiding presence of YESHUA THE MESSIAH.

When HE is acclaimed and has sovereignty in the soul there is purity, bondage is smashed and delivers freedom from sickness and disease. Victory enters our lives and even though we pass through the canyon of death we know HE is there to encourage us by HIS WONDROUS LOVE for HE carries our burdens and revitalizes us when we call upon HIM.

The glory, fullness and completeness of HIS gospel plan can be fulfilled within our life with our acceptance of HIM. We will have perfect peace, complete love and abundant assurance. The beauty and the fragrance of HIS Character will shine as a Standard of benevolent love and a signatory to the world that we are HIS.

Our countenance, our walk and our fruit will reflect YESHUA as others are captivated by the glory of an abiding MESSIAH. As others see the reflection of YESHUA through us many will desire HIM in their life. Like a magnet they will be drawn by the Magnificence of HIS Light shining through HIS devoted family as glory overflows back to the Great Giver of life in currents of praise and thanksgiving

There is nothing GOD desires so much as witnesses who will represent HIS SPIRIT and CHARACTER and there is nothing this world needs worse than the manifestation through humanity of the SAVIOR'S LOVE. All Heaven is waiting for channels through which can be poured the Holy Oil to be a joy and blessing to human HEARTS for healing and salvation.

Even so from GOD'S Righteousness to self-righteousness is but a small distance and our balance lies only in GOD'S SPIRIT proven through GOD'S WORD.

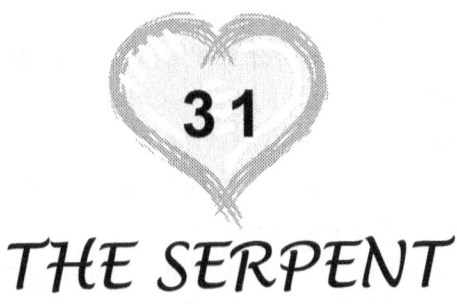

THE SERPENT

The suggestion that sin is extinguished apart from the law brings to mind the serpent lying inactive and motionless, hidden as if dead in the garden waiting for the opportunity to leap into life and cause havoc. Nothing resembles an expired serpent more than an active snake as it lies quietly, as if asleep. Therefore we can not yield to comfort and take for granted the murderous stick of the attacker, nor can we venture into the enemies establishments of sin without being attack unless we go in concealed in GOD'S protection and for HIS purpose.

The unseasoned believer is apt to come under attack by satan the serpent due to the newness of their belief and lack of knowledge of GOD'S SACRED WORD, for sin is like a striking serpent or a military strategist that has made GOD'S Law a base of operations. Iniquity turns GOD'S BLESSING, the law into a curse by deception and fraud and those unwilling to search GOD'S WORD and study to be approved are most vulnerable to satan's wicked pranks of evil. The Law was perverted by sin and made subservient to its treacherous works of doom but GOD'S divine intention is for Law in it's truest form to reveal and expose sin.

To absorb GOD'S WORD is beneficial for us because the soul that is uninformed of the prohibition of the law is intoxicated in unrecognized sin; but when the knowledge of sin comes it will cause repentance or it will justify self to arouse rebellion against the Law, which reserves the right to continue in the 'THOU SHALT NOTS' which permit iniquity to achieve all kinds of covetousness where sin is glorified, personalized and personified.

Man's intellectual teaching has replaced GOD'S, not only in the substance of nature, but in sacrificial service. The SCRIPTURE given to reveal GOD has been so perverted until today they have become the means of concealing HIM.

YESHUA'S teachings have lost their meaning as men lack focus to discern GOD in HIS Works. The sinfulness of humanity has launched a shadow over the impartial face of creation; until now instead of manifesting GOD, HIS works have become a barrier that conceal HIM.

ROMANS 1:25b Men "WORSHIPPED AND SERVED THE CREATURE MORE THAN THE CREATOR". Thus the heathen :21b 'BECAME VAIN IN THEIR IMAGINATIONS, AND THEIR FOOLISH HEART WAS DARKENED." {depressed-oppressed-surpressed mental states}

YESHUA did not deal in abstract theories, but in the essential development of a perfect HEART, excellent health and good character. These commodities are priceless and will enlarge man's capacity to know GOD and increase the human efficiency for good.

YESHUA is the spokesman for truth that correlates the conduct of life with good health and springs from a pure HEART. These are the possessions that take hold upon eternity relative to the commandments and ordinances of HIS FATHER. For it is the laws and principles of GOD'S kingdom that reveal soundness of mind and body as well as the elegance and cherished abundant life. Even so to acknowledge and accept this wisdom is the privilege each is granted by GOD'S Grace and encapsulates the freedom to chose good or evil, YESHUA or satan. We can not accompany, satisfy or obey both. To know YESHUA we must seek HIM in HIS WORD. Nonetheless we are born unto sin, therefore the activities of the flesh come natural but to solicit our own desires is to cultivate the germ of sin that gives promotion to satan.

Mankind has fallen prey to the world system where satan the serpent is the satanic god, who sets those up for a fall who are occupied with the pride of their accomplishments through self exaltation. In not knowing or understanding that the 'alien sin' enters the body for total destruction and only the Divine Physician YESHUA can remove that 'hostile offender' to secure a new HEART and abundant life. GOD created each of us, put our human system in place, and consequently it is no problem for our CREATOR to heal and cleanse us from sickness and disease or even death.

A few insightful physicians of this generation have began to observe GOD'S WISDOM and have recognized the prudence of good thinking v. bad thinking, joyful attitude v. bad attitude, truth v. evil. They are beginning to understand the extraordinary effect the be-attitudes have in our lives but if, in their advancement of good knowledge, they reject YESHUA, they will remain empty and void of discernment and saving knowledge.

Few doctors' have confidence in GOD'S WORD where all pragmatic and beneficial wisdom is concealed. In their refusal to depend upon GOD they deny the proven fact that when the SCRIPTURE is examined, cherished and exercised it will automatically produce excellent health of mind, body, spirit and HEART. THE SCRIPTURE relays vast remedies for wellness and the one most urgent is 'BE HOLY', seek to make HIS Will the desire of the HEART, emulate HIS Holiness and as a result walk in perfect health to experience a little bit of Heaven here on earth.

There is not anything unattainable with GOD WHO knows each and every hair on our head and divinely placed every vessel, muscle, cell, bone, nerve, etc., in the exact place so as to organize a divine service to our body and then gave to us HIS DIVINE breath that contributes the very oxygen that we breathe.

We acquire everything out of the possessions of GOD yet when we are ill we transfer our trust from GOD to a man of flesh, who is unable to create a vessel, muscle, cell, bone, nerve, etc., and has no authority except to bind up, transplant, remove from, replace a part from another body or foreign object. But in essence he has no ability to heal, assign us life or death, except that we give him or he usurps.

YESHUA linked HIS teaching not only with healing but also with the day of rest and the week of toil. HE gives wisdom to him who drives the plow and sows the seed. In the plowing and sowing, the tilling and reaping, HE teaches us to see an illustration of HIS work of grace in the HEART. So in every line of useful labor and every association of life, HE desires us to find a lesson of Divine Truth. As we reach a point of submission to GOD our daily toil will no longer absorb our attention and lead us to forget HIM; it will continually remind us of our CREATOR and REDEEMER. The thought of GOD will run like a thread of gold through all our homely cares and occupations. The glory of HIS Face will again rest upon the expression of nature. We shall ever be learning new lessons of heavenly truth and growing into the image of HIS purity. For we shall 'BE TAUGHT OF THE LORD", and in the lot wherein we are called, we shall "ABIDE WITH GOD". {Is. 54:13; 1 COR. 7:24}

We must daily reinforce ourselves with the mind of YESHUA by absorbing HIS WORD which will provide the will and the power to put to death the sin nature in self-denial. If we choose the way of the stubborn and rebellion all sympathy and tenderness for YESHUA our MESSIAH is lose by omission and we become mockers. Thus the adversary comes in as a roaring lion to devour and claim the soul as naked territory, he begins an assault with deadly weapons upon the mind, tempting the intellect with ungodly ideas draped in fun and excitement prepared to lead us into wrongdoing and lasciviousness.

EPHESIANS 6:16 ALWAYS CARRY THE SHIELD OF TRUST, WITH WHICH YOU WILL BE ABLE TO EXTINGUISH ALL THE FLAMING ARROWS OF THE EVIL ONE. JEWISH NEW TESTAMENT

YESHUA'S Blood Shed is our armor of assurance, our spiritual defense from satan and when we are in the Will of GOD we walk in an anointed and divine place. Even when satan torpedoes his darts of sin into our mind GOD'S salvation is at work to provide protection. The only fear of satan is the Blood of YESHUA that defeated him at Calvary.

The initiation of all disgrace originates in the HEART not in sacrament or calamity upon the body. The acceptance of THE WORD will make a phenomenal alteration in the HEART and life, it will alter the disposition and dialogue of all who encounter.

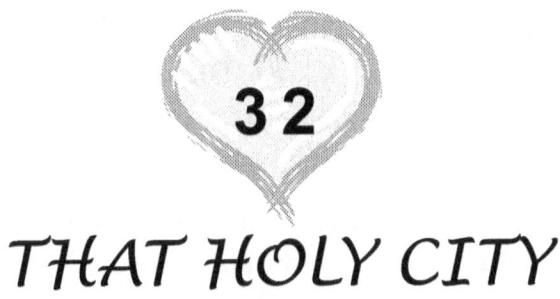

THAT HOLY CITY

REVELATION 21 reveals a Holy City in the New Jerusalem that will come down to exhibit the Blessed presence of GOD. All tears will be wiped away by the Heavenly Father, there will be no more sorrow, pain, nor crying. The truth and certainty of this blessed estate are ratified by the WORD and the promise of GOD.

Our walk on earth is merged with a sad mixture of corruption and grace but upon entrance to the Holy City we will be cleansed by the laver of YESHUA'S BLOOD and presented to the FATHER without spot. Everyone will be equal, there will be no one impure, we will dwell for all eternity in a perfect and pure society.

REVELATIONS 22 extols Heaven as Paradise where there will be abundant love, delight, glorious peace and happiness. We will experience springs of grace, comfort and glory in GOD flowing through YESHUA. Its quality pure and clear as crystal with a tree of life fed by pure waters from GOD'S Throne, wholesome fruit is available that provides health and happiness. We will be sealed by GOD in a place where there is no evil for all eternity.

YESHUA sought to eliminate that which obscures truth. The veil that transgression launched over the face of nature HE draws aside as HE brings to view the spiritual glory that all things were created to reflect. HIS WORDS placed the teachings of nature and the BIBLE in an unspoiled aspect to make them a fresh revelation as HE awarded us power and authority over demons.

LUKE 9:1 CALLING TOGETHER THE TWELVE, YESHUA GAVE THEM POWER AND AUTHORITY TO EXPEL ALL THE DEMONS AND TO CURE DISEASES; AND HE SENT THEM OUT TO PROCLAIM THE KINGDOM OF GOD AND TO HEAL. JEWISH NEW TESTAMENT

YESHUA empowers us today just as HE armed the Disciples of HIS day with power and authority over demon spirits, to dispose and cast them out. HE also authorized and appointed HIS Followers to cure disease and heal the sick. These gifts were a part of their commission and have neither been taken back or stopped. Even so vain traditions coupled with the self-righteous pride of men down through the ages, who have called themselves teachers of GOD but in essence have brainwashed many who are today unable to understand YESHUA is the resurrection for all time, for yesterday, today and forever. GOD is still the Great Physician and Healer and HE still issues omnipotence from HIS Royal Seat to accomplish the supernatural through those who donot doubt HIM today.

All who spurn HIS healing ability, HE invokes as HE did the men who were with HIM in the boat when the great storm arose "OH YE OF LITTLE FAITH".

GARDEN OF THE HEART

The HEART is a garden that must be cultivated. The impenetrable boulder that has crusted many times over has created layers of rock that have made the HEART inaccessible and insensitive. This bedrock must be crushed in earnest repentance of iniquity, for this explosive rock, although hardened by rebellion and rejection runs the risk of bursting under pressure. But in the meantime it will block the passage of blood that is life to the body and will cause skepticism that is deadly to any HEART because unbelief always hinders any healing that has already been paid for by YESHUA at Calvary.

Poisonous, satanic seed that has taken ground and matured into disease and plague must be uprooted and the nearer we draw to YESHUA the light, the darkness where pain and disease hides must flee. Consequently the soil overgrown by thorns can be reclaimed by diligently seeking the LORD. Thus the evil tendencies of the natural HEART can be overcome only by earnest effort in the Name of YESHUA. HE has told us in HIS WORD through HIS prophet to:

JEREMIAH 4:3 BREAK UP FALLOW GROUND AND SOW NOT AMONG THORNS{SIN}. HOSEA 10:12 SOW TO YOURSELF RIGHTEOUSNESS; REAP IN MERCY. JEWISH TANAKH

When we believe in and submit to YESHUA through obedience, HE consummates a desire in the HEART to obey HIM by seeking HIS WILL. We enthusiastically become sowers of HIS seed with an fervent zeal and passion, telling others how wonderful HE is as we display HIS forgiveness and GODLY affection. We are excited about the change we have witnessed in our own life as well as others and long to prepare the HEART of everyone we know or meet for HIS GOSPEL by gently leading or being an example of HIS LOVE. Our faith, trust and walk with GOD, when in earnest will cause others to hunger for the element of peace and strength that we display in our life. They too, will be willing to come boldly to the LORD and take possession of the Gospel as we did and that will break the chains of bondage the enemy now binds them with.

Unfortunately satan is more familiar with GOD'S WORD than most believers, and this corrupt one dispatches his demon colleagues in haste. These brute spirits arrive on the scene arrayed with SCRIPTURE and go into the streets of Christendom, orphanages, institutions, hospitals, homes, and anywhere he can slither his way into, for the specific purpose of luring all those who are suffering with an empty spot in their HEART, that do not realize that YESHUA paid the supreme price for their freedom.

These freakish spirits of corruption deliver the lost and confused into enslavement through bondage. They seek out those who reject the MESSIAH, who refuse to allow GOD to influence their life through HIS WRITTEN WORD. In their unwillingness to pursue THE LORD the doorway to their HEART is thrown open for the prince of darkness to gain entry for the exclusive intent of disaster. Upon arrival of the demoniac spirit{s} the individual egotistically attacks others to mimic the devil and trails satan's demon angels into the trap of the abyss. We must all be warned that satan's singular resolve is to steal, kill and destroy {John 10:10}.

AMERICA'S CUP

THE BALANCE OF JUSTICE WEIGHS HEAVE

AMERICA'S CUP IS FILLED WITH SIN

INNOCENT BLOOD SCREAMS FROM THE GROUND

GREED AND PRIDE ARE GROUND WITHIN

SODOMITES SCREAM FOR EQUAL RIGHTS

AS DO WOMEN WHO ENVY MEN

OUR COURTS ARE MADE UP OF PETTY FOOLS

THAT HEAP LIES ON MOUNTAINS OF SIN

THEY CLOSE THEIR EYES AT NIGHT TO DREAM

OF VICTIMS THAT THEY HAVE WRONGED

NOT UNDERSTAND THEIR FUTURE TO BE

TO REAP EACH VERSE OF THE SONG

WHILE CHURCHES ARE OPEN

TO THE PIOUS THAT BE

WHO CALL THEMSELVES CHRISTIAN

SET IN DAZED APATHY

NOT CARING FOR THOSE THAT

HE DIED TO SAVE

WITH THEIR BLOOD ON OUR HANDS

THEY GO TO THEIR GRAVES.

His mother called him Yeshua, the world calls him Jesus

This generation has emphasized their vigilance on lecturing sermonettes, building pew numbers and the tithe which is to frequently for the advancement of human goals, the HEART is taken for granted and given only petty regard. The urgency for the REDEEMED to cultivate the souls of the destroyed and befuddle persons with acts of devotion and prayer is overwhelming. Just as YESHUA demonstrated sympathy and mercy for the imperfect and decaying life we must pray for GOD to prepare our HEART to minister to them and prepare their HEART to accept our message about THE LORD.   Pray that GOD draws others into SALVATION and that HIS HOLY SPIRIT inspires and stimulates their attention toward the majestic gift of eternal life and smothers them with good deeds and affection from those who love as HE loves..

Even though the HEART is as cruel as the beaten highway and it seems as if our efforts are useless we must present the SAVIOUR of the GOSPEL to all; even when logic fails and explanation seem powerless to convince, the love of YESHUA revealed in personal ministry will relax the stony HEART and cause a grain of truth to root. If we have the melody of faith in our HEART it will be heard by the look on our face.

GOD does not judge a leader by the numbers that are led but by those who genuinely encounter spiritual growth in the HEART. A sower of HIS WORD will be affectionate and faithful to illustrate the sympathetic commitment of YESHUA expressed in compassion. The Believer will be a radiant model in demonstration to reach others through conduct and disposition in relation to them, so that the seed may not be strangled with thorns or perish because of shallowness of the soil.

MATTHEW 13:18 SO LISTEN TO WHAT THE PARABLE OF THE SOWER MEANS :19 WHOEVER HEARS THE MESSAGE ABOUT THE KINGDOM BUT DOESN'T UNDERSTAND IT, IS LIKE THE SEED SOWN ALONG THE PATH - THE EVIL ONE COMES AND SEIZES WHAT WAS SOWN IN HIS HEART. :20

THE SEED SOWN ON ROCKY GROUND IS LIKE APERSON WHO HEARS THE MESSAGE AND ACCEPTS IT WITHJOY AT ONCE. :21 BUT HAS NO ROOT IN HIMSELF. SO HE STAYS ON FOR A WHILE; BUT AS SOON AS SOME TROUBLE OR PERSECUTION ARISES ON ACCOUNT OF THE MESSAGE, HE IMMEDIATELY FALLS AWAY. :22 NOW THE SEED SOWN AMONG THORNS STANDS FOR SOMEONE WHO HEARS THE MESSAGE, BUT IT IS CHOKED BY THE WORRIES OF THE WORLD AND THE DECEITFUL GLAMOR OF WEALTH, SO THAT IT PRODUCES NOTHING. :23 HOWEVER, WHAT WAS SOWN ON RICH SOIL IS THE ONE WHO HEARS THE MESSAGE AND UNDERSTANDS IT; SUCH A PERSON WILL SURELY BEAR FRUIT, A HUNDRED OR SIXTY OR THIRTY TIMES WHAT WAS SOWN.JEWISH TANAKH

The different types of seed {persons} described in the above SCRIPTURE who become familiar with THE GOSPEL are the casual{V.19}, the shallow{V.20}, the worldly{V.22} and the responsive {V.23}. The seed is the same; the soils are different. Consequently a 'mixed community' is developed, caused by the SON of MAN sowing good seed and the devil sowing weeds. In the end the truth will be revealed and men will be divided into two classes, the evildoers who will be rejected by GOD or the righteous who will radiate the glory of HIS acceptance.

Often troubles are the tools which GOD uses to fashion us with for better things even so there is always opposition from the attacker and the world, both in tribulation and persecution and in its cares and pleasures. The SOWER can be sure that although most of the seed is wasted the harvest will be abundant.

Since our DIVINE CREATOR chose to structure each one special there are diversified models of humanity and each will experience different calls to the GOSPEL. Our choices are the hinges of destiny. The depth that we connect with "GOD'S WORD" will adjust in harmony with our earnestness to lay hold and concentrate our attention to "IT". By confirming all instruction we are given by man in GOD'S WORD we will experience great wisdom and strength. For there is more safety with THE MESSIAH in the tempest than without THE MESSIAH in the calmest waters.

PSALMS 121:7-8 THE LORD WILL KEEP YOU FROM ALL HARM, HE WILL WATCH OVER YOUR COMING AND GOING BOTH NOW AND FOREVERMORE. N I V

The HOLY SPIRIT keeps vigilant watch on the HEARTS of men and when HE finds a HEART that is deserving and cleansed HE inserts new significance for the GOSPEL within the mind and life takes on new meaning. Our excitement ponders amid GOD'S family with enthusiasm and we begin to examine HIS WORD, THE BREAD OF LIFE from the KING of KINGS, LORD of LORDS. Giver of life eternal and our inspired magnetism becomes contagious.

If we are reluctant to examine and analyze SCRIPTURE, the serpent is prepared to swoop down like the buzzard to snatch any ineffectual WORD we have been exposed to. Just as the devil did to Eve in the Garden of Eden as he focused on the crisis of faith and unbelief. He coiled THE WORD into a lie and turned man's GOD-given probationary opportunity into an avenue of temptation.

The stipulations of GOD'S Covenant Law had been challenged by the deceiver himself as he related to Eve 'YOU WILL BE LIKE GOD'; satan had re-interpreted GOD as a devil, a liar possessed by jealous pride and re-established the way of the curse as the way to blessing.

Adam and Eve were condemned by their own terror. Just as many today are convicted in the HEART when the Divine Judge looks down upon their HEART. The reaction of this SEAT OF PASSION reveals the truth and anticipates the verdict but GOD cuts through this subterfuge, exposing the act of disobedience as the root of evil. By self-justification we challenge the CREATOR in arrogance and therefore annihilate our own well being.

The angel fetched Peter out of prison, but it was prayer that fetched the angel {Thomas Watson}. We must be faithful to abide in prayer with anticipation, with our eyes primed to weep so that our head does not swell with pride. Lest we become so occupied with ourselves that YESHUA can not be seen or perform through us. We must inquire and retain firmly the foundation principles of HIS WORD so that at all times we will display HIS Character and be prepared to carry on even under the affliction of others. Capable and willing to deny natural inclinations and endure as a good soldier.

PSALMS 119:30 I HAVE CHOSEN THE WAY OF FAITHFULNESS; I HAVE SET YOUR RULES BEFORE ME. JEWISH TANAKH

MATTHEW 22:37 LOVE THE LORD YOUR GOD WITH ALL OUR HEART AND WITH ALL YOUR SOUL AND WITH ALL YOUR MIND. NIV

Whatever a man loves is his god. For he carries it in his HEART. {Martin Luther}. We must determine by faith to trust in YESHUA so completely that it will radiate in our life and our joy will be established in winning souls for HIM. When we learn to profile this kind of lifestyle to the condemned world they will witness YESHUA through our life.

Demonstration of HIS love from the HEART will cause others to desire HIM and pleasures of the world will surrender their power and attraction. The plowsharing of truth will break up fallow ground, cut off the top of thorns and pull the weeds [of sin] by the root to replace them with grapevines of HIS GLORIOUS WORD. Seeds of health and wisdom will vault from the HEART and the HOLY SPIRIT will step forward to glorify GOD and give us new abundant life filled with HIS joy and grace.

1 CORINTHIANS 13:4 LOVE IS PATIENT AND KIND, NOT JEALOUS, NOT BOASTFUL :5 NOT PROUD, RUDE OR SELFISH, NOT EASILY ANGERED AND IT KEEPS NO RECORDS OF WRONGS. :6 LOVE DOES NOT GLOAT OVER OTHER PEOPLE'S SINS BUT TAKES ITS DELIGHT IN THE TRUTH :7 LOVE ALWAYS BEARS UP, ALWAYS TRUSTS, ALWAYS HOPES, ALWAYS ENDURES :8 LOVE NEVER ENDS; BUT PROPHECIES WILL PASS, TONGUES WILL CEASE, KNOWLEDGE WILL PASS :13 BUT FOR NOW, THREE THINGS LAST, TRUST, HOPE, LOVE; AND THE GREATEST OF THESE IS LOVE. PURSUE LOVE. JEWISH NEW TESTAMENT

It is the charitable HEART not the voluble tongue that is acceptable to GOD. A clear and wise head is of no significance without a benevolent and charitable HEART for it is not immense knowledge that GOD sets value upon, but authentic and HEARTY affection and love. Miraculous mountain moving faith in HIM does not account to HIM as much as does the loving charity of the HEART. True charity is the HEART and SPIRIT of SALVATION and if the sacred heat of love is not coupled with charity and embedded in the HEART it is of no profit, and worth nothing.

GOD requires us to fill the mind with good and pure thoughts. HE urges us to meditate upon HIS Love and mercy and study HIS phenomenal actions in the immense scheme of redemption. As we surrender to HIS WILL our perception of truth, desire for purity of HEART and clarity of conviction become superior and virtuous and our healthy existence will be strengthened because our HEART will be rewarded.

The soul dwelling in the safe atmosphere of holy anticipation will be transformed by communion with GOD through the study of the SCRIPTURES, thus we will fully-develop and BRING FORTH GOOD FRUIT in obedience.

Upon acceptance of YESHUA we thwart satan's passage for damnation where all who reject HIS love and mercy will go to scorch forever and forever and forever and forever and forever. For the unsaved: GOD removes HIS Protective covering and allows satan to take authority. 'The enemy' quickly advances and begins to torment the mental balance until the affliction is so burdensome that the mentality is enslaved and violated under the stress.

Even than GOD sends others along side to warn the wonderer or backslider, in an attempt to make straight the way back to SALVATION. The message is given in love and patience and the ALMIGHTY will not permit one to mock HIM, HIS DIVINE CHARACTER OR HIS SON. So if the adverse soul rejects the warning{s} and remains rebellious, it will be captured by satan and thrust head long into evil preparing to meet HIS CREATOR only to be denied the eternal Heaven. He will be rushed right on into hell.

JAMES 1:22 DON'T DECEIVE YOURSELVES BY ONLY HEARING WHAT THE WORD SAYS, BUT DO IT!

JAMES 2:26 INDEED, JUST AS THE BODY WITHOUT A SPIRIT IS DEAD, SO TOO FAITH WITHOUT ACTIONS IS DEAD.

There are three stages for a believer as he begins his journey into faith, first the conscience is informed and believes by faith. Secondly belief and faith are exercised and third, GOD's will by the Fire of the HOLY SPIRIT inspires the HEART with a burning desire to serve thus we spring into action. The WORD is often compared to a mirror for it shows a man himself as he is and the sight is not pleasing because the WORD will reflect the inner HEART. Moral insides and aspirations will convict the conscience which speaks to the HEART and will cause the HEART to become new if heeded, or will cause the HEART to become hardened if rejected. Thus the unity of the body and spirit aptly point to the unity of faith and works.

EVIL DEEDS

Because the sinner is not punished immediately they begin to assume their evil will not be found out, that perhaps GOD does not see or somehow excuses them. With that mind set they resist GOD'S law and in defiance their HEARTS are full in them to do evil; they venture to do more mischief, and commit iniquity with a high hand to bring about curses of sickness and death upon their families and themselves.

But sentence is passed against evil works and evil workers by the righteous JUDGE of heaven and earth and the execution is often delayed, even so sinners have deceived themselves for though the sentence is not executed speedily, it will be executed more severely at last.

ECCLESIASTICS 8:11 THE FACT THAT THE SENTENCE IMPOSED FOR EVIL DEEDS IS NOT EXECUTED SWIFTLY, WHICH IS WHY MEN ARE EMBOLDENED TO DO EVIL JEWISH TANAKH

35

HEARTS of STONE

Hardness or hardening of the HEART is directly connected to our relationship with GOD and is the reason for HEART attacks, HEART disease, etc. The HEART is the intermost center of the natural condition of man and bodily life, the reservoir of the entire life power. GOD'S WILL is synonymous with fullness, wellness, abundant life. HE is the faithful protector and enforcer of moral law, no one can be excused nor hidden from HIM and HIS Covenants are established more firmly than the pillars of heaven or the foundation of earth and cannot be dis-annulled. It is an honor and a favor to be employed for and used by HIM in doing good. On the other hand a wicked man's days are all as a shadow, empty and worthless. Any peace or joy the wicked know or have will be short lived for even their memory will perish and be over when this life on earth comes to the end. The life on earth will be counted for little if remembered at all and eternity will be spent in the misery and pain of the fiery pit.

MICAH 6:13 THEREFORE WILL I MAKE THEE SICK IN SMITING THEE, IN MAKING THEE DESOLATE BECAUSE OF THY SIN.

When we give thought or action to satan he comes in as a flood and slowly begins to cover and blind us, satan will cultivate our world with evil if we allow him into our HEART. But when we belong to GOD, the enemy can only enter our world when we move away from GOD. Our problems appear when we walk out of HIS WILL and anything that does not please GOD or is out of HIS WILL is of no value and a by product of the enemy.

TO LIVE BY FAITH

For over a year Noah built the ARK out of obedience, he pleaded with those of his time to repent before he went into the ARK that he and his family had built, but the world stood around laughing at them. It was Noah's submission of obedience to GOD'S command and Noah esteemed GOD above those of the world. He continued to do GOD'S WILL. As he worked and continued telling others in the world about eternal life and we too, must plead with others to repent as we build our ARK in obedience by faith and good works of charity.

Noah gave up his home, land and possessions by faith to GOD'S Command in "obedience". What ever was competition to GOD'S WILL, Noah disregarded as he submitted to the confinements and inconveniences of the ARK in order to preserve his family and himself in SALVATION for the new world. He denied himself and his pleasures both in suffering and service in order that he could provided life for his family through his walk with GOD at the ARK.

HEBREWS 11:7 BY TRUSTING, NOAH, AFTER RECEIVING DIVINE WARNING ABOUT THINGS AS YET UNSEEN, WAS FILLED WITH HOLY FEAR AND BUILT AN ARK TO SAVE THIS HOUSEHOLD. THROUGH THIS TRUSTING, HE PUT THE WORLD UNDER CONDEMNATION AND RECEIVED THE RIGHTEOUSNESS THAT COMES FROM TRUSTING. JEWISH NEW TESTAMENT

It was after the land had dried and the family came out of the ARK to begin in celebration of GOD'S deliverance, new life and the vineyard that Noah over indulged in wine to be come drunk and pass out in a stupor. That is when Ham's act of malicious disrespect gave evidence to the serpents seed in the remnant family.

Noah's drunken condition caused him to lay bare and the exposure of his nakedness recalls satan's work in Gen. 3. The covering of nakedness by two of Noah's sons recall the divine covering of fallen man by the Blood of animals, which pointed to a future reference of YESHUA'S covering of Blood for our sin and a spirit devoted to the imitation of GOD.

The Old Testament [Covenant] points us to works, the law by which no man can keep or have salvation. It was literal mankind written on stone for external law. The new Testament [Covenant] is inward, written on the HEART and points to mercy coupled by Divine Love in spirit, truth and obedience from the HEART. The New Covenant is symbolic of the Old Covenant with the condition set in the HEART instead of stone, with the will and the conscience of each as a part of GOD'S own family, HIS Will becoming our will as we draw nearer to HIM in obedience, HE administers our new HEART.

JEREMIAH 31:32,33 IT WILL NOT BE LIKE THE COVENANT I MADE WITH THEIR FATHERS, WHEN I TOOK THEM BY THE HAND TO LEAD THEM OUT OF THE LAND OF EGYPT, A COVENANT WHICH THEY BROKE, I WILL MAKE WITH THE HOUSE OF ISRAEL AFTER THOSE DAYS, DECLARES

THE LORD; I WILL PUT MY TEACHING INTO THEIR INMOST BEING AND INSCRIBE IT UPON THEIR HEARTS. THEN I WILL BE THEIR GOD, AND THEY SHALL BE MY PEOPLE.

As GOD shut the door of the ARK for Noah and his family's protection, HE will shut the door of our ARK [symbolic] for our protection, the world will laugh at us for our salvation, as they refuse to listen. But when we are truly HIS and understand what awaits those who jest and make fun, our HEART will be wrenched in grief ready to plead for their forgiveness, as we become willing to say "FORGIVE THEM FATHER FOR THEY KNOW NOT WHAT THEY DO". However even though they continue to laugh in their season of fun and laugher, we must continue to build our ARK, witnessing to soul upon soul, nailed together by the demonstration of our walk and talk in GOD'S grace and mercy. We will reflect the MASTER as we dwell in charity, love, peace and mercy toward others. Just as HE pours HIMSELF out to us so we must pour ourselves out to others in HIS Divine agape love and charity.

Our endeavor to reflect Our MASTER, to pour ourselves out to others must be authenticated in HIS DIVINE LOVE from the depth of forgiveness and compassion of our HEART. If a GOD like compassion or love is not felt than we deal in idolatry and self-righteousness thus our labor is of no significance and our effort may cause more harm than help. As we attempt to lead in love, we must also be willing to step aside and allow the HOLY SPIRIT to go into the HEART and harvest GOD'S WORD that we have hopefully planted.

JOHN 14:26 BUT THE COUNSELOR, THE RUACH HAKODESH [HOLY SPIRIT], WHOM THE FATHER WILL SEND IN MY NAME, WILL TEACH YOU EVERYTHING; THAT IS , HE WILL REMIND YOU OF EVERYTHING I HAVE SAID TO YOU. JEWISH NEW TESTAMENT

As we prepare for the ARK we must bring all those who are willing to enter by good instruction, persuasion and good example and be in readiness to guide them gently by assisting them through prayer to destroy their death clothes {dirty garments, baggage of the world} not from self righteous zeal lest we forget that we too, came from that world of unbelief driven by demon spirits. Death clothes are the ugly baggage we accumulated in the world such as attitudes, resentments, temperament, indignation, bitterness and the like.

For an unbeliever to come to YESHUA will involve a revolutionary alteration of will and regeneration of the HEART, the Divine gift. A HEART that knows and expresses GOD discerns instinctively and does spontaneously what GOD requires, and by faith knows that only GOD is the giver of New HEARTS.

JEREMIAH 24:7 AND I WILL GIVE THEM THE UNDER-STANDING TO ACKNOWLEDGE ME FOR I AM THE LORD. AND THEY SHALL BE MY PEOPLE AND I WILL BE THEIR GOD, WHEN THEY TURN BACK TO ME WITH ALL THEIR HEART. JEWISH TANAKH

With the HEARTS radical change will come forgiveness of all past sin. Old scores will be wiped away and a new beginning will issue great advancement to a higher realm. The relationship to GOD will become immediate and direct and will flow as a life of harmony with GOD'S PERFECT WILL and will be reflected through our works.

GOD is HOLY, and HE has made holiness the moral condition necessary to the health of HIS body as well as HIS universe. Whatever is Holy is healthy; consequently evil is a moral sickness that must end ultimately in death.

Moral health is a by-product of faith in GOD, whatever is contrary to GOD'S WILL brings GOD displeasure and to preserve HIS creation GOD will destroy it or in essence, allow satan to captivate it and satan's only goal is to "STEAL, KILL AND

DESTROY" JOHN 10:10. The very word Holy is derived from the Anglo-Saxon halig, hal, meaning well, or whole.

JEREMIAH 31:34b I WILL FORGIVE THEIR INIQUITIES AND REMEMBER THEIR SIN NO MORE. JEWISH TANAKH

The mark of one who walks in SALVATION is demonstrated in all manners of speech, ability and actions because to walk with the LORD is wisdom. All who are not found in YESHUA {JESUS} WHO is the ARK of DIVINE PROTECTION, are undone and should be pitied because their eternity will be spent in hell. We must be careful to love and pray for them but not careless in our association to condone or cherish their ways lest we fall into the same pit prepared by the adversary.

If we are careful to hold up GOD'S Standard, speaking as a reflection of HIS Love and SALVATION, by HIS anointing power we will be judges of evil in demonstration of wisdom and power. With out speaking a word our countenance will glow and be glorified as evil is condemned. For in HIS Divinity only, we are equipped to break the chains of bondage that satan binds with.

The bondage of evil, like cords will hold the captive under satan's power until YESHUA is allowed in to take over, for only YESHUA defeated the attacker and only HE can break all bondage placed upon us by the enemy.

SIN

1 PETER 2:5 YOU YOURSELVES, AS LIVING STONES, ARE BEING BUILT INTO A SPIRITUAL HOUSE TO BE COHANIM {HIGH PRIEST} SET APART FOR GOD TO OFFER SPIRITUAL SACRIFICES ACCEPTABLE TO HIM THROUGH YESHUA THE MESSIAH. JEWISH NEW TESTAMENT   GENESIS 4:7 SURELY IF YOU DO RIGHT, THERE IS UP LIFT. BUT IF YOU DO NOT DO RIGHT SIN COUCHES AT THE DOOR;

ITS URGE IS TOWARD YOU, YET YOU CAN BE ITS MASTER.
JEWISH TANAKH

Sin is synonymous with sickness, sorrow, suffering, etc., it is a demon spirit who couches and waits for any one passing, to leap upon and devour. As it bullies its way in to the HEART it is fully set for destruction. To STEAL, KILL AND DESTROY. JOHN 10:10. It is so contagious that when we co-mingle with one whose conscience has been seared, who commits willful and flagrant sin and has defiled their system to walk in evil, we stand in danger of polluting ourselves. Lest we speak with a sorrowful HEART for the state of their soul and eternal destiny, we are not a reflection of YESHUA but rather our salt has lost its flavor, our message is useless and we speak in pride promoting our fleshly wisdom of GOD'S WORD.

YESHUA is the ONE - WHO gave HIS LIFE and HIS love is a love of mercy for all, from the lowest life to the king and we have no righteousness accept through HIM. When we judge sin and speak in pride, we set ourselves up as god, to seek idol worship and idolatry that is looked upon by GOD as adultery. By idolatry we prostitute our salvation with falsity and our spirit becomes polluted for only the MESSIAH is our alter and the true Tabernacle.

HEBREWS 8:2 THERE HE SERVES IN THE HOLY PLACE, THAT IS IN THE TRUE TENT OF MEETING, THE ONE ERECTED NOT BY HUMAN BEINGS BUT BUILT BY ADONAI [THE LORD]. JEWISH NEW TESTAMENT

Through YESHUA, GOD dwelled among us and it is through YESHUA that our sacrifice of obedience is acceptable to GOD, donot be deceived for SALVATION and Divine Health is in and by YESHUA only.

The conscious mind is a spark of the almighty GOD and has a powerful effect upon the health. Our subconscious is to often at the root of our condition because thought is a force, even as electricity or gravitation that will draw us away from GOD into our own selfishness. So too, will our stinkin-thinking give cause to dis-ease and plague. We can hear our conscious mind reason with our HEART but are often unaware of our subconscience mind, it's power and persuasion can make us weak or strong. That is the reason we must guard what is fed into our mind, through our eye.

JOB 11:20 BUT THE EYES OF THE WICKED PINE AWAY; ESCAPE IS CUT OFF FROM THEM; THEY HAVE ONLY THEIR LAST BREATH TO LOOK FORWARD TO. JEWISH TANAKH

To often we are guilty of causing our own illness by refusing to let go of a thing that we harbor. Soundness of mind and body is something we want as long as it doesn't interfere with 'the thing' we want more. The fervor for health is secondary such as one who desires recovery from emphysema but the craving is second to the death defying lust to smoke, thus the illness is self inflicted. In effect it is sin against the body, the temple. Our rewards will be according to our obedience.

Then there is the alcoholic who desires healing of the affliction but without giving up the bottle or the overweight person who wants healing of obesity and hardening of the arteries but refuses to diet and exercise or even give up all the junk foods that cause the problems.

While the inner voice screams from within and disposes of money to investigate healing the subconscience repudiates any effort to give up the objective, the root obstacle. So the damage is allowed, even encouraged to grow.

Sometimes the difficulty is financial and produces distress [stress, dis-ease] that develops friction in the spirit and points to future disease or HEART problems. Still we can't stop spending money we don't have so we withdraw from changing our life style for fear of loosing status, and the pride of life makes us harder and drives us into a corner, surrounded by financial woe, causing our HEART to fear or even fail.

When all we need to do is back up, give up, submit to and let GOD run our lives. HE has a way of making us comfortable, giving us pleasure in the real things of life that count such as peace and joy with our family. Keeping us satisfied with what we have, not grasping for more "things" that neither live or breath nor care if our grasp for them causes our death.

PROVERBS 13:15 GOOD SENSE WINS FAVOR; THE WAY OF TREACHEROUS MEN IS UNCHANGING. JEWISH TANAKH

Often our pain stems from a broken relationship, a fuss, disagreement, divorcee or even death. GOD handles even those hurts and pains if we let HIM and we will come out wiser, stronger and healthier if we just give it all to GOD, HE will carry us.

There are numerous reasons for illness and no one, not even the good physician comprehends the logic of our bodies afflictions, but GOD does and HE has all the answers. Illness is usually the outer expression of a deep and possibly dangerous struggle within our HEART. Occasionally unsuspecting illness may be a method of coping with a predicament that we are powerless to hold up under or put up with, therefore sickness, accidents and tragedy could all be the senseless option of choice to release repulsive realities. When cinched by a daily dilemma it may be lowliness or arrogance that keeps us from backing away to get a good prospective on the situation for a necessary change but no modification will make a difference without GODLY wisdom as our leader.

When we attempt change without the LORD involved it is a temporary cul-de-sac. One of shallowness with no lasting effect, heading for another of societies contemporary, yet short lived solutions.

In The Meaning of Persons, Dr. Tournier says "A very real and painful migraine, a distressing liver attack, or a stubborn diarrhea may manifest themselves every time one has to deal with a difficult situation. People who are hard of hearing have confessed to me, too, that they have sometimes been grateful to their infirmity for allowing them to evade an unwelcome dialogue".

In essence sickness and impairment may be an unconscience means of securing love and attention we believe we cannot obtain in any other way. A child is a good example when they pretend sickness to keep from attending school to perhaps miss a test or a bad experience with one of their school mates or perhaps just needs some special love and attention from mom at home.

In many cases we will find people refusing unconsciencely, they are unwilling to give up their conditions or illness because in a perverted way they need their sickness to draw others to them in sympathy. Often they give up the opportunity for mature loving relationships for the sake of controlling a situation in the only way they understand, by commanding love and attention in a way they learned in their childhood either by watching another control others, or perhaps their own control of always seeking and obtaining what they want. What a sad way to gain attention or exist, in a vacuum of control.

Perverted pride paraded as weakness will cause life to be dependent up on others, to cling as a vine that chokes out any real living, exploiting misery. How tragic that so many depend upon and become accustom to sickness and misery as if they are fearful of freedom, when all they really need is GOD in their life for wholeness.

We are exercising hopelessness, making amusement and even mocking GOD when we diddle with or attempt to manipulate others by our frustrated and perverted mind set, it is an evil from the pits.

OCEAN OF SIN

Values challenged, sin creeps in

Immorality as white caps, hit the shore and blend

The tide now has covered, us and the shore

Seduced by the tide of perversion, as we sat in a state of ignore.

We stand up in amazement, looking of someone to blame

Covered with sin and corruption, this is no longer - just a game.

The flood of evil and wickedness, crept in as a thief

How did it start? Where did it come from?

satan and his deceit.

Even so, the Blood of YESHUA can destroy the captivity of perversion and free us from enslavement if we will allow HIM to take control. HE will not only give us liberty but issue a new HEART occupied with the beneficial possessions necessary to render life and eternity in a perfect HEAVEN

It is a blasphemous condition of mind that says LORD, my sin is bigger than YOUR forgiveness, my weakness and my sickness is greater than YOUR power to heal, my problems are to big for YOU to solve. At that point we have become wrapped in our own finite misgiving of "me" or "my" and the big "I" of self confidence has blinded us to GOD'S infinite power, production, love and mercy.

Sin can utterly acquire dominion over a believer just as soon as we walk out of GOD'S WILL if we yield premise to mischievous thinking, evil works and the like. But even as we sin, if we realize our status of authority in YESHUA, we can petition forgiveness of our sin with HEART felt devotion and vow not to repeat whatever transgression we had executed, and be installed again on the

His mother called him Yeshua, the world calls him Jesus

moral avenue of forgiveness by the LORD because we are under the Blood of YESHUA.

Let us not at all be convicted of thinking there is another way of forgiveness or salvation than the Blood of YESHUA because any other method is a cult and is considered sin in GOD'S EYES, fit for destruction in the bottomless pit of fire.

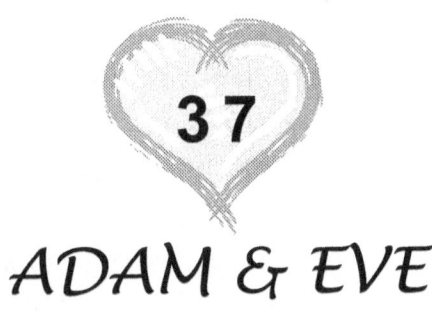

ADAM & EVE

Our sin was born in Eden when, with one stroke satan reinterpreted GOD as a devil, a liar filled with jealous pride. Eve was deceived into thinking the way of the curse was the way of blessing, thereby diverting attention from the spiritual direction of man's likeness to GOD, the tempter satan reduced the issue to merely a formal existential matter of ascent to god-hood. When Eve consented to satan's theology, anti-faith was birthed.

But GOD made provision for those who draw near to YESHUA to give rise to restitution for sin, find for-giveness, healing, favor and eternal life through the SON, YESHUA for a HEART restored.

Adam and Eve were created by GOD in innocence and placed in a perfect environment, subjected to a simple test. They were warned of the consequences of disobedience. Adam was not compelled to sin for he knew no sin before that time but he was tempted, just as we are tempted today by satan as Adam was we have a choice to obey or disobey.

1 TIMOTHY 2:14 IT WAS NOT ADAM WHO WAS DECEIVED, BUT THE WOMAN WHO, ON BEING DECEIVED, BECAME INVOLVED IN THE TRANSGRESSION. JEWISH NEW TESTAMENT

Eve was deceived but Adam transgressed deliberately and with that disobedience, the test was failed, the stewardship of innocence ended in judgment of expulsion from Eden, removed from GOD'S Divine Garden into a world where satan is god.

This was the Divine Magna Charta for all true scientific and material progress as GOD in HIS anger for Adam's disobedience destined all mankind to a shorter life span and subjection to satan's taunts.

GENESIS 3:24A GOD DROVE THE MAN OUT AND STATIONED EAST OF THE GARDEN OF EDEN THE CHERUBIM AND THE FIERY EVER TURNING SWORD, TO GUARD THE WAY TO THE TREE OF LIFE. JEWISH TANAKH

GOD had given mankind a mind of perfection in its finite capacity for learning and from that mind all was perfect and good, where evil was hidden and unknown.

Mans purpose was to subdue, acquire a knowledge and mastery over the material environment and bring all elements into the service of the race. God had Covenanted with Adam as HE made a sovereign pronouncement to establish a relationship of responsibility between HIMSELF and Adam.

What a wonderful place we could live in today had Adam and Eve not been tempted of satan, the enemy serpent. Just as with Adam, HE Covenants with us today and expects a relationship of responsibility in faith and righteousness from the HEART to bring elements that we control into service for HIM and reflect HIM in that service. We too, can [symbolically] walk in that Divine place until we allow the enemy to tempt us and choose to follow. At that point we step into satan's domain with out GOD'S Divine Protection.

The stipulations of GOD'S Covenant laws were challenged by satan and as a result the senses of Adam and Eve became a physical shame. The serpent's council had manifested consciousness of inner nakedness, stripping the glory of holiness from their soul. Their home where GOD had placed them was a Garden, a Holy Place and man's position there involved priestly vocation and obedience but Adam failed, much like many of us fail daily to live in harmony with GOD'S WILL and become deceived or deliberately and purposely transgress.

Adam was educated by GOD and forbidden to eat of the tree of good and evil but in his plight to please his mate he humbled himself by allowing Eve to take a leadership position and give him "fruit" from the tree in disregard and disobedience to GOD'S Will. Today we to, as Adam did, are guilty of seeking to please man rather than GOD.

There was no trial for satan, he was sentenced because the LORD of the Covenant had instituted HIS lawsuit against the unfaithful and Divine Justice could not be denied, thus GOD drove man from the Garden and set guards up to protect the Sacred Garden and the tree of life.

When Adam and Eve ate the fruit and wrongdoing became a state of being, they realized their nakedness and guilt immediately caused their shame as they attempted to hide their embarrassment with fig leaves but GOD seen their HEART. HE knew they had disobeyed, just as HE knows our every thought and intent of our HEARTS and judges each according to the HEART attitude.

The awareness of shame attached to the physical nakedness manifested mindfulness of their inner exposure as it stripped the distinction of holiness from their soul. In anxiety they fashioned for themselves aprons from fig leaves to mask their guilt as if that would be a refuge from GOD in HIS own sanctuary. Their own terror condemned them, for in such an ordeal of confrontation with the divine Judge the HEART'S reaction reveals the truth and anticipates the verdict.

Adam's sense of nakedness was like his fear, an evil consequence of his rebellion for GOD had cut through the deception, exposing the act of disobedience as the root of evil. The sinner avoided confession of guilt only by the blasphemous expedient of virtually blaming GOD for his fall as he told GOD "THE WOMAN WHOM THOU GAVEST".

Eve too, sought to absolve herself from blame by pointing the finger at the serpent. Therefore GOD cursed the serpent to slither in the dust, subject to trampling and the serpent became a symbol of humiliation and condemnation.

Because the ground was entered into the composition of man [MADE FROM DUST] the curse on the ground became a power unto death working in his very members. Death, formerly present in nature in subservience to man but would now terrorize man the covenant-breaker as the wages of his sin.

The redemptive victory would involve suffering thus GOD symbolized HIS purpose to restore men to fellowship with HIM in the provision of the act of animal sacrifice. The sinner's shame, as a religious problem, could not be covered by their own efforts and animal sacrifice was set in place as a temporary covering pointing to the ultimate and final sacrifice of YESHUA'S PERFECT AND PRECIOUS BLOOD.

PSALMS 66:18 HAD I AN EVIL THOUGHT IN MY MIND, THE LORD WOULD NOT HAVE LISTENED.   JEWISH TANAKH

The BLOOD of YESHUA will forgive us of all our confessed sins, but will not cover even one of our miserable excuses nor the fig leaves we attempt to take refuge in. An animal had to die so that Adam and his wife might be clothed. Here we find the first example of the great Biblical Doctrine, the innocent dying for the guilty.

GOD established the animal offering for sin in the Garden of Eden as HE poured forth the life's blood of an animal to camouflage the nudity of Adam and Eve for the fig leaves were inadequate. Never the less Adam and Eve instituted a pattern that mankind has continued to use down through the ages as they sew fig leaves together in a puny effort to disguise their sin. The fig leaves are in the form of good works, church attendance, giving money for worthy causes, etc., somehow in the minds of many the fig leaves justify and cover shame.   But the guiltiness in our HEART can not be concealed from GOD and as "IT" is exposed it obligingly maligns the health where strife, pain, hardness of HEART and even death begin to take root. As GOD covered the nakedness of Adam and Eve, blood sacrifice was birthed to glorify GOD in acknowledgment that all man's provision is from HIM and to verify that all men are sinners.

YESHUA was predetermined to be the conclusive BLOOD Sacrifice for all transgression but today's environment observes nakedness as a element of glorification to gleam and lust after. Many have lost vision of GOD as their sense of right and wrong stands as a monument to shame and sex as dishonor parades in our streets and our homes throughout the Nation. satan has so encircled us with evil corruption much due to the laziness and cowardliness of "believers" whose salt has lost it savor and the era has reached a point where the everyday fashion event is a naked body. We have become so desensitized to evil that we are now unequivocally wasted by our laxed-nonchalent attitude.

ISAIAH 5:20 AH, THOSE WHO CALL EVIL GOOD AND GOOD EVIL; WHO PRESENT DARKNESS AS LIGHT AND LIGHT AS DARKNESS; WHO PRESENT BITTER AS SWEET AND SWEET AS BITTER.   JEWISH TANAKH

Those of the world who see our precious MESSIAH must see that our sacrifice is in obedience by faith to acknowledge that all we have is from GOD and that we are all sinners and come far short of HIS GLORY. We should not engage in fantasies nor become vein about service for GOD lest we become mockers and set ourselves up as our own god. In our pretense of honoring GOD, we have dishonored HIM.

DIVINE INSTITUTION

GOD meant marriage to be a divine establishment of commitment between man and woman, who was taken from his side [the rib]. Fully intended for comfort in human life and the decent and honorable propagation of the human race. Such as became the dignified behavior of man's nature above that of the beast.

GOD'S code for marriage is that two become one flesh. By marriage there is equality in man and wife founded in consent and custom. Any other form of marriage as in same sex, incest, etc., can not be justified but adds guilt of profaning the ordinance of GOD and prostituting marriage to the vilest of purposes which was instituted for the noblest ends. Uncleanness committed with any other outside of marriage is forbidden and is the reason GOD has deemed any different type of union as a sin deserving death for it places evil intents upon a sanctified and holy union instituted by GOD HIMSELF.

Entrance of sin is the instrument of satan who turned GOD'S given probationary opportunity into an avenue of temptation.

Eve yielded to usurped authority but Adam completed the fall in his disobedience, thus sin and death were passed to all men.

ROMANS 5:12 HERE IS HOW IT WORKS; IT WAS THROUGH ONE INDIVIDUAL THAT SIN ENTERED THE WORLD, AND THROUGH SIN, DEATH; AND IN THIS WAY DEATH PASSED THROUGH TO THE WHOLE HUMAN RACE, INASMUCH AS EVERYONE SINNED. JEWISH NEW TESTAMENT

In the Old Testament, blood sacrifice was obligatory and performed once a year for the sin of all people. However with the New Testament Covenant, YESHUA became that BLOOD Sacrifice for the iniquities and infirmities of all. It was for our transgressions that HE willingly submitted to shed HIS perfect Blood at the Cross to became our sacrifice. Our obedience to HIS WILL is captivated in our profession of HIM and is gained by a repentant HEART. In return for obedience HE gives assurance of eternal salvation and divine protection as we sojourn in mundane existence and remain steadfast in HIS peace, joy, love. HE has provided the Sword of HIS SPIRIT through HIS WORD for our protection and it is our duty to keep that Sword sharp by going daily into HIS WORD to be equipped with HIS weapons of warfare against satan, which is HIS SCRIPTURE.

The rudiments of this world, though we may or may not be squarely set to see them are to be tutors of testing, to prepare us to be wise and sanctify ourselves so that we may learn to be Holy. If GOD be Holy, we must also strive to be Holy, else we cannot expect to be accepted by HIM. GOD sent us HIS ONLY SON, a SAVIOUR WHO came to free us from our sin, washed us white as snow and gives us a new HEART. A HEART that will desire to do HIS WILL, it is up to each of us to accept HIM with the whole HEART, to fight the good fight and to manage wrong desires by refusing to look or be involved in the evils of our society.

There is always a price to pay. When the BIBLICAL STANDARDS of morality give way to dishonesty and deceit,

GOD will send calamity and disaster to the HEART of those who refuse to repent and it will begin slowly with benign signs of stress, fatigue, anxiety, unforgiveness, envy, judgment, doubt, distrust, fear, worry, pessimism, discouragement, frustration, impatience, prejudice, arrogance, ungratefulness, selfishness, and a clinging to material things that have no life of their own, but have become items of worship. One becomes prideful thinking they have achieved and are above others and cannot be bothered or touched. Therefore exaltation results.

With the acceptance of these disruptions in one's spirit the FIRST GREAT COMMANDMENT has been abandoned for it declares THOU SHALT have no other "gods" for HE is a jealous GOD, full of holiness and justice WHO will not allow HIS creation to make sport of HIM nor to stand prideful before HIM.

CORINTHIANS 11:2 FOR I AM JEALOUS FOR YOU WITH GOD'S KIND OF JEALOUSY; SINCE I PROMISED TO PRESENT YOU AS A PURE VIRGIN IN MARRIAGE TO YOUR ONE HUSBAND, THE MESSIAH.

JEWISH NEW TESTAMENT

Nature is content with little, grace with less but lust with nothing. We have left HIS WILL to demand after our own cravings and satan's ambush will seduce us into slavery and cause disgrace, sickness, disease, and dishonor. Our insides have firmly incorporated the big "I" in the foreground of GOD'S predetermined will for our life as we demand our own carnality. Sin has side tracked human inventiveness down a frustrating remedial road and we have moved away from GOD'S DESIGN, not vice-versa.

GOD'S WORD directly associates to the individual and every fragment of our lives, our being and our body; but we are incompetent to realize that unless we recognize HIM and willingly surrender to HIS WORD in repentance with a faithful passion to change from the HEART.

PSALMS 40:8 I DESIRE TO DO YOUR WILL OH MY GOD, YOUR LAW IS WRITTEN IN MY HEART.

When that deep repentant spirit becomes an objective we will hunger for all HE offers. Our desire will be to read HIS WORD regularly, to study, consume and abide by it.

HIS SCRIPTURE is to be our illustration of prudence and instruction. It is our option to conform to HIS WILL or go our own direction that is fashionable where we chase human culture. As we stride 'our own way' we must bear in mind that satan is the god of this world and as satan's subjects we are destined to be stolen from, killed and destroyed. John 10:10

One of the most urgent, over looked and ignored problems of society today, is the spiritual corruption of the HEART. For from the HEART comes all the issues of life. We have the ability to make choices of what to do and which Master we will follow. If we choose satan, we will be the instrument of satan's torment and eventual defeat but if we choose YESHUA we become the instrument for satan's defeat through our authority given us by OUR LORD.

If satan can acquire our HEART he can also monopolize our life and the options we make will give birth to curses in the lives of our children and their children and so on to the third and fourth generation. Unless of course they turn from the prince of darkness to seek the light of YESHUA.

EXODUS 20:5 YOU SHALL NOT BOW DOWN TO THEM OR SERVE THEM. FOR I THE LORD YOUR GOD AM AN IMPASSIONED GOD, VISITING THE GUILT OF THE PARENTS UPON THE CHILDREN, UPON THE THIRD AND UPON THE FORTH GENERATIONS OF THOSE WHO REJECT ME, :6 BUT SHOWING KINDNESS TO THE THOUSANDTH GENERATION OF THOSE WHO LOVE ME AND KEEP MY COMMANDMENTS.

GOD will not penalize the children for the fathers' sin unless they perpetuate the same violations or when the sins committed involve certain social and physical consequences. Those who will be punished are those who 'hate' GOD but HIS mercy transcends HIS wrath, and HIS blessing are upon those who love and obey HIM and they will reach into a thousand generations.

Be sure that GOD will not relinquish what is HIS equitable due in terms of reverence and obedience to be bestowed upon anything else. HIS honour is anchored by HIS children's worship attendance and is a manifestation of GOD'S righteous character.

The accomplished impostor, satan has centuries of experience in bewitching and perverting souls into hell. He has the expertise to fabricate all the things that we cherish just as we wish, and will bait us at our weakest point and make it gratifying, full of life, lights of glitter, great fun, and seemingly innocent but after a while what ever is not of GOD will be empty and ugly. For all of satan's inner workings are superficial, disastrous and corrupt. Without warning we will notice ourselves 'out on a limb', all alone again but instantly satan gives birth to a new smoke screen to ensnare us one more time. All of a sudden we are elevated to the loftiest stratosphere causing us to indulge our cavalier conceit once again only to be ostracized in the end with disappointment and grief, full of emptiness. Another merry go round of glittering lights one more time, left alone.

If we grow exhausted in regard to hearing about repentance it's because there is an urgency to repent. If we are weary of hearing about deliverance, it's because we need it. If we are worn out about hearing about finances, that's a sure indication that there is no generosity in our HEART.

LOOK! WHO IS THAT?

If YESHUA walked into the majority of organized religions today, HE would be abruptly ushered out and ordered to depart from the premises. HIS ministry was unconventional, HIS techniques are inappropriate according to our sophisticated, intellectually oriented lifestyles. YESHUA brazenly associates with sinners, dishonest tax collectors and known prostitutes and is not confined or inhibited by prohibition or pressured by popular opinion. HIS apparel would scandalize the majority and HIS Standard of HOLINESS would irritate most of the leaders.

The "tradition of men" make GOD'S WORD of none effect, as ears of today hustle about tuned to tradition and the words of men. We have allowed mans image to obscure the true image of YESHUA'S reflection to create a death producing tradition of men.

MARK 7:6 HE ANSWERED AND SAID UNTO THEM, WELL HATH ESAIAS PROPHESIED OF YOU HYPOCRITES, AS IT IS WRITTEN, THIS PEOPLE HONOURETH ME WITH THEIR LIPS, BUT THEIR HEART IS FAR FROM ME; :7 HOWBEIT IN

VAIN DO THEY WORSHIP ME, TEACHING FOR DOCTRINES THE COMMANDMENTS OF MEN :13 MAKING THE WORD OF GOD OF NONE EFFECT THROUGH YOUR TRADITIONS, WHICH YE HAVE DELIVERED; AND MANY SUCH LIKE THINGS DO YE.

Even so, GOD is always there to meet us where we are, whether it be in the ditch or on the throne, HE'S our safety net at the end of a lonely trail and HE will gather us when we are on bottom and love us unconditionally. It is sad that in the majority of "Churches", believers set peacefully in a comfort zone and are not bothered with those who wonder about on the streets for fear of getting their hands dirty. They refuse to spread the good news about YESHUA and how HE died for all. They refuse to give a hurting person a place to find solace, to mentor them in the ways of GOD, HIS LOVE, the freedom HE gives and the ever lasting life available for all in HIS SCRIPTURE.

As we begin to examine and literally embrace what GOD says is true, we begin to be convinced and realize that GOD'S WORD does not return void. We find it quite simple to understand that everything we say and do with our own free will has a direct effect upon every member of our body, especially the HEART because that is where all the issues of life stems from. HIS WORD will make us radical as we are inspired by HIS POWER to lay anointed hands on sick bodies, cast demons out of tormented individuals, tell others about the GOSPEL of HIS KINGDOM fervor and passion and pray - pray - pray for GOD tells us in:

LUKE 6:45 A GOOD MAN, OUT OF THE GOOD TREASURE OF HIS HEART, BRINGETH FORTH THAT WHICH IS GOOD; AND AN EVIL MAN, OUT OF THE EVIL TREASURE OF HIS HEART, BRINGETH FORTH THAT WHICH IS EVIL; FOR OUT OF THE ABUNDANCE OF THE HEART HIS MOUTH SPEAKETH.

The magnificent system GOD placed into each body, made in HIS Image was planned for HIS pleasure. Since HE is Perfect in all HIS ways, it only makes good sense that HIS creations would begin as 'perfect'.

A radical believer is not measured by great feats of religious activity coupled with pride, but is measured by simple obedience. Fear of being labeled "radical" has prevented many from rising to meet the need and assuming their rightful position in spiritual authority. The threat of controversy has caused them to draw back from truth. We say we will obey the WORD of GOD as long as it doesn't involve the word "GO" or "PRAISE HIM IN THE SANCTUARY", for fear of raising our arms in front of other men who may criticize or make jest of us.

PSALMS 107:31 OH, THAT MEN WOULD PRAISE THE LORD FOR HIS GOODNESS, AND FOR HIS WONDERFUL WORKS TO THE CHILDREN OF MEN :32 LET THEM EXALT HIM ALSO IN THE CONGREGATION OF THE PEOPLE, AND PRAISE HIM IN THE ASSEMBLY OF THE ELDERS.

Our faithfulness and obedience to GOD signifies our thankfulness to HIM for HIS mercy, protection and HIS gift of eternal life. When we sin and return to HIM with our HEART full of repentance and thanks for HIS mercy, HE is quick to forgive. But let none of us think for any reason that GOD requires no service from us for HE plainly tells us: "MY CHILD, GIVE ME THY HEART" and when we do that HIS HOLY SPIRIT employees us for service to HIS WILL.

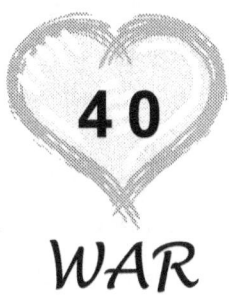

WAR

Whether we recognize it or not we are a victim in the midst of warfare for our soul which began at birth. Even as GOD gives the gift of a child to a parent, satan grandstands near by, eager to attack and destroy. This war is waged by the monarch of hell who intends to penetrate and monopolize each of us to demoralize and poison our system, so that we are not only prepared for hell but we will recruit others for this firey eternity. This war is spiritual and begins in the conscience to cause us to mock and doubt GOD but GOD is supreme and refuses to be mocked.

GOD places a shield of protection around those who are HIS and Heavenly Angels stand on every side. But HIS DIVINE protection is only for those who choose wisdom over insanity and will begin reading and studying HIS BOOK OF LIFE. Otherwise we walk in darkness, unable to discern tricks and attacks of the enemy, as our souls are invaded, seized, assaulted and violated on every side often with no chance of recovery. The attacker is pragmatic about destroying our mind and our HEART is so covered with walls, hardened with no defense yet with no way out.

We must determine to train our thoughts and restrain our mind from the dominion of sinful affections and dispositions which cause disease and defilement. Our preparation for diabolical warfare is described through strategic meditation of SCRIPTURE and consummated by diligent prayer and thanksgiving so that we are able to stand against satan and rebuke his wares as they enter the eye on the way to the HEART. We will be diligent to reprove satan by our discernment of GOD'S WORD.

Our doubt about GOD enters when our 'free will' over rides HIS WILL as we commence to exalt 'self'. We move forward in self-righteousness to become our own god and in self worship we refuse GOD'S Will for our life and follow our own fleshly desires. Our words and wisdom have filled us with arrogance and cast a clumsy screen across the consistent pattern of GOD'S plan for us.

We should be zealous to take possession of GOD'S WORD, to listen to the preachers and teachers who fear and cry and pray for our life. To listen with an open mind so that the HEART no longer rejects HIM, WHO is our SAVIOUR. The rejection of restorational truths in the Body of YESHUA must come to an end. Times demand that we be weaned from the milk of the WORD to strong meat, subjected to the higher authority of GOD'S WORD.

HEBREWS 5:12 FOR ALTHOUGH BY THIS TIME YOU OUGHT TO BE TEACHERS, YOU NEED SOMEONE TO TEACH YOU THE VERY FIRST PRINCIPLES OF GOD'S WORD ALL OVER AGAIN. YOU NEED MILK, NOT SOLID FOOD. :13 ANYONE WHO HAS TO DRINK MILK IS STILL A BABY, WITHOUT EXPERIENCE IN APPLYING THE WORLD ABOUT RIGHTEOUSNESS :14 BUT SOLID FOOD IS FOR THE MATURE, FOR THOSE WHOSE FACULTIES HAVE BEEN TRAINED BY CONTINUOUS EXERCISE TO DISTINGUISH GOOD FROM EVIL. JEWISH NEW TESTAMENT

Just as satan exalted himself and was thrown from Heaven, many of us have exalted ourselves and stepped out of GOD'S protection to be subjected to satan's bondage of sin, shame and sickness.

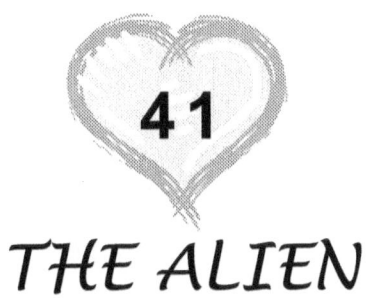

THE ALIEN

When sin and rebellion enter into the Divine System GOD has given to us, it is alien to GOD'S purpose. Our system doesn't understand how to deal with that alien incorrect input. Our system doesn't grasp and can not find a slot or a place for sin so it has no choice but to send 'sin' to the HEART, the BOSS where all issues are settled. In trying to deal correctly with the alien sin, the HEART in confusion begins to reject and grow hard and begins a slow process of failure, of death.

The sin spirit is from the adversary and it arrives with one design in mind and that is destruction. GOD'S original purpose for the HEART was sinlessness. It was not meant to be subjected to or know evil therefore the HEART can not accept this 'alien evil' as a part of GOD'S equipment so the HEART begins a hardening process and little by little it begins to crust over and over until it becomes completely hardened and diseased from the results of sin coming in like a flood.

PSALMS 40:12 FOR TROUBLE WITHOUT NUMBER SURROUND ME; MY SINS HAVE OVER TAKEN ME AND I CANNOT SEE. THEY ARE MORE THAN THE HAIRS ON MY HEAD AND MY HEART FAILS WITHIN ME.

THE UNBELIEVER V. THE BELIEVER

Characteristics of the human heart are challenged every second as many great minds of this time lean toward the atheistic theory of evolution which holds that man is accidental and a random product of a blind and nonpersonal series of chemical and biological events. This theory would have us believe that our world and all it contains came into being through evolving mud in time past. An unscriptural and nonsensical theory that has taken this world by storm due to the apathy and unbelief of many confirmed believer. Can we not wonder if they believer at all?

When we possess faith, we move about and make use of that which we have confidence in. Such as our car, if it is a worthy automobile we sat in it and turn the ignition key in faith that it will start. We take journeys in it with assurance that it will transfer us to our destination. Faith is just believing and using the means of that belief to accomplish an end, depending on what our desired end is.

Let us assume GOD is a brand new-fashioned automobile and "IT" is ours to use as we wish. If we are fully confident and believe "IT" is capable of carrying us where ever we wish to go, we will move about with surety of its ability and power.

Our assignment is to make sure "IT" is properly serviced such as:

1} daily gas fill {reading GOD'S WORD daily}

2} tune up {being among others who love HIM as often as possible}

3} gauge check {keep HEART tender before GOD}

4} keep good tires on road {travel in peace, love, joy, reflecting YESHUA}

5} keep it clean {prayer alone and incorporated}

6} keep inside clean {watch our tongues, refrain from gossip}

The difference is our dependency is not on any man made item such as a car but in the ALMIGHTY for GODLY Faith is believing in the OMNIPOTENT BEING, WHO will move mountains when we are faithful and obedient to HIS WILL.

When we are HIS CHILDREN and confident of HIS power we will know beyond the shadow of any doubt that GOD is the answer for all things. Be it health, healing, marriage, children, family, safety, job, transportation, travel, food, clothes, etc. What ever is our need HE has the Divine competence and energy to deliver within the framework of HIS PRESENCE with joy unmeasurable, peace in the midst of the storm, entwined with complete happiness. Each of the above named functions and many more that we can not comprehend are as significant to HIM as they are to us because they are befitting for us, but none are as urgent to OUR HEAVENLY FATHER as our eternal life consequently as HIS children, HE spanks us when we are naughty and rewards us when we are faithful.

Unfortunately most of today's population who claim to be believer's use GOD as if HE were an old broken run down automobile and they doubt HIS ability to sustain them or that HE will even start {hear them}. So they promenade in fear, apprehensive about HIS Power to repair {heal}. Therefore most have turned to the physician, the ways of the world first instead of taking their problems to the ALMIGHTY for complete and comprehensive healing of the mind, body, and soul. Most consider HIM as antiquated, aged and unable to operate in such a wicked world and HIS omnipotence and competence has somehow been bound up in Heaven with HIM. As long as they refuse to believe in GOD'S POWER, HE is unable to work in their lives.

Eventually due to our tired, weak and pesky attitude of pain and worry, our wonderfully created system begins to clog. Glitches come as irritation and our foundation begins to wobble as we become nervous and stress sets in. We become unable to deal with normal problems that in good health would be only a passing thought.

The door to our soul has opened because of problems, complaints and worries. Hence satan enters, seeking to steal, kill and destroy and his destiny is total destruction.

JOHN 10:10 THE THIEF COMES ONLY IN ORDER TO STEAL, KILL AND DESTROY; I HAVE COME SO THAT THEY MAY HAVE LIFE, LIFE IN ITS FULLEST MEASURE. JEWISH NEW TESTAMENT

Why do we not realize that we were made in GOD'S Image of HIMSELF. It is we who have failed HIM because our mind has sought 'self' fulfillment? We are unprepared and blinded without GOD, and have no understanding of sin and rebellion for it is the enemy within each of us. It comes in alien spirit form and we have no control, for only GOD has power over the enemy spirits. But in our self seeking, we have become blinded to HIS WILL as we grope about in anger and bitterness, complaining that HE pays no attention to our needs and does not care. The fault lies within us who have sought to close HIM out of our lives to 'do our thing'.

Yet we, when seeking our selfish will are unaware that we open the doors for enemy spirits to make an entrance and penetrate our soul as slowly we turn from GOD unto sin and walk after our own lust.

Do we now expect GOD to rescue us, to send angels into the temple of our body to disarm and put the enemy within us out? Even though HE is a forgiving GOD, HE will not force HIS way. However HE will dispatch spirit Angels to snap us without hesitation from the sinister clutches of the attacker if we call upon HIM in deep HEART felt repentance

2 CORINTHIANS 2:11 LEST satan SHOULD GET AN ADVANTAGE OF US: FOR WE ARE NOT IGNORANT OF his DEVICES.

When we first begin to turn our back on GOD our tender consciences becomes less sensitive by every compliance to evil. One sin prepares for another, even pleads for it by making it necessary for concealment.

Every step forward to satan's ground deprives us of the secure promises of GOD and binds us to agony that will causes our soul's distress and deliver pain and disease. Since the beginning of time satan has attempted to destroy, mock and deceive any thing GOD created and called good. Since satan, the enemy can not get to GOD he continually comes against GOD'S most precious creation which is the HEART of mankind.

Attacked, bound and blinded by this monarch from hell, mankind has stumbled and turned from walking in GOD'S Will that will shower GOD'S blessings to 'satan's' calamity as he strives without exception to profane and bind us beneath his suppression just as he did with Adam and Eve in the Garden of Eden, when he mocked GOD'S flawless marriage between man and woman as he twisted GOD'S truth. Just as he continues in his hideous diabolical fashion to beguile mankind today by producing seeds in judgment of others that cause us to suppose our own self righteousness and consider that we are intelligent enough to channel our own conscious with out GOD.

ROMANS 1:22 CLAIMING TO BE WISE, THEY HAVE BECOME FOOLS. :23 IN FACT, THEY HAVE EXCHANGED THE GLORY OF THE IMMORTAL GOD FOR MERE IMAGES, LIKE A MORTAL HUMAN BEING, OR LIKE BIRDS, ANIMALS OR REPTILES. :24 THIS IS WHY GOD HAS GIVEN THEM UP TO THE VILENESS OF THEIR HEARTS' LUSTS, TO THE SHAMEFUL MISUSE OF EACH OTHER'S BODIES. :25 THEY HAVE EXCHANGED THE TRUTH OF GOD FOR FALSEHOOD, BY WORSHIPPING AND SERVING CREATED THINGS, RATHER THAN THE CREATOR, PRAISED BE HE FOREVER. AMEN :26 THIS IS WHY GOD HAS GIVEN THEM UP TO DEGRADING PASSIONS; SO THAT THEIR WOMEN EXCHANGE NATURAL SEXUAL RELATIONS FOR UNNATURAL; :27 AND LIKEWISE THE MEN, GIVING UP NATURAL RELATIONS WITH THE OPPOSITE SEX, BURN WITH PASSION FOR ONE ANOTHER, MEN COMMITTING SHAMEFUL ACTS WITH OTHER MEN AND RECEIVING IN THEIR OWN PERSONS THE PENALTY APPROPRIATE TO THEIR PERVERSION :28 IN OTHER WORDS, SINCE THEY HAVE NOT CONSIDERED GOD WORTH KNOWING, GOD HAS GIVEN THEM UP TO WORTHLESS IMPROPER THINGS :29 THEY ARE FILLED WITH EVERY KIND OF WICKEDNESS, EVIL GREED, AND VICE; STUFFED WITH JEALOUSY, MURDER, QUARRELING, DISHONESTY AND ILL-WILL; THEY ARE GOSSIPS, :30 SLANDERERS, HATERS OF GOD; THEY ARE INSOLENT, ARROGANT AND BOASTFUL; THEY PLAN EVIL SCHEMES; THEY DISOBEY THEIR PARENTS; :31 THEY ARE BRAINLESS, FAITHLESS, HEARTLESS AND RUTHLESS, :32 THEY KNOW WELL ENOUGH GOD'S RIGHTEOUS DECREE THAT PEOPLE WHO DO SUCH THINGS DESERVE TO DIE; YET NOT ONLY DO THEY KEEP

DOING THEM, BUT THEY APPLAUD OTHERS WHO DO THE SAME. JEWISH NEW TESTAMENT

Even so humanity still makes an effort to camouflage and defend immoral intents in their good works, self proclamation, self righteousness, etc., thinking GOD can not see the wretchedness and hardness of the evil in our HEART. How absurd we are for such self- admiration. We are subjected daily to the tree of good and evil as we walk in this world and most embrace evil in rebellion, not understanding or even being concerned that the avenue of temptation is the pathway to death.

Our character displays our moods of behavior and issues ultimate destinies. When our aspiration are righteous, our faith in ONE GOD maintains our protection through promises in HIS WORD. Our righteousness does not indicate sinless perfection but the resolute cast of our mind that we are determined to be different and <u>are not governed</u> by the same ideas as the wicked. We organize and scrutinize our time and are cautious about what enters our eyegate and we are careful to examine our feelings in GOD'S WISDOM because YESHUA has given us the authority and wisdom through HIS BLOOD to flee from bondage.

PHILIPPINES 2:5 LET YOUR ATTITUDE TOWARD ONE ANOTHER BE GOVERNED BY YOUR BEING IN UNION WITH THE MESSIAH YESHUA. JEWISH NEW TESTAMENT

GOD does not reap wrath where HE does not sow knowledge. But for one to consider that he might be acquitted on the premise of illiteracy is preposterous for all men have both the witness of conscience and that of nature. These twin witnesses are unmistakable and universal. As a result all men are exposed both to them and by them. For man to deny GOD and look with in himself is deemed self-righteous and they generally make one of two mistakes. They misunderstand the height of GOD'S law or they underestimate the depth of their own moral conduct.

They desire the fruit of Christian blessings but refuse the origin of it's.foundation as they ignore or disregard the awesome knowledge of GOD. It was GOD WHO set the stars in place and knows their number. It is GOD WHO knows man's thoughts and directs his steps. It is GOD WHO looks upon the HEART. It is GOD WHO knows the number of hairs on each head. It is GOD WHO knows the past, present and the future and it is all in the PALM of HIS MIGHTY HAND.

When we sanctify our aim to obey in harmony and become firmly established in the LORD our pleasure will emphasize and focus upon HIS WILL. For to do righteousness was set forth in HIS Divine plan and the voice of HIS HOLY SPIRIT speaks to us through the still small voice {conscience} to influences our HEART for encouragement or warning. The conscience is equipped with the knowledge to know right from wrong, it is a birth right, delivered to the HEART upon our creation, in HIS Image.

ROMANS 2:15   FOR THEIR LIVES SHOW THAT THE CONDUCT THE TORAH [LAW] DICTATES IS WRITTEN IN THEIR HEARTS. THEIR CONSCIENCES ALSO BEAR WITNESS TO THIS, FOR THEIR CONFLICTING THOUGHTS SOMETIMES ACCUSE THEM AND SOMETIME DEFEND THEM. JEWISH NEW TESTAMENT.

Faith has been defined as 'the hand of the HEART'. Thus by faith we must reach for GOD'S Gospel to sustain our sojourn here. In HIS WORD we find HIS POWER that produces HIS Righteousness that will elevate us to a superior horizon then that of the world and although we walk on every side of the world we are not in it. Somehow we are detached and even capable of observing the intensity of curses that others, who do not know the LORD provoke, to imprison themselves in slavery to the adversary.

The word Righteousness simply defined, means 'right clothing' and we all must be clothed rightly to receive HIS Blessings. The

SCRIPTURE tells us that all sinners are naked before GOD. Some sinners realize this and attempt to make their own suit of spiritual clothes but GOD looks upon such clothes as filthy rages {Isa 64:6}. However GOD provides new clothes from HIS GOSPEL to all repenting sinners. GOD is righteous, HE demands righteousness and HE provides righteousness. But GOD'S fierce wrath is revealed against all ungodliness {sin against HIS PERSON} and unrighteousness {sin against HIS WILL}.

GOD'S nature is unchanging and hostile to all that offend HIS Righteousness. HE estimates each of us by our moral standards and HE discounts a reprobate mind. GOD refuses to hear the prayer of a rebellious, self righteous sinner who mocks HIM and HIS wonderful gift of life through HIS SON without repentance.

ROMANS 1:28 AND EVEN AS THEY DID NOT LIKE TO RETAIN GOD IN THEIR KNOWLEDGE, GOD GAVE THEM OVER TO A REPROBATE MIND, TO DO THOSE THINGS WHICH ARE NOT SEEMLY.

HIS WORD plainly states that by HIS death at Calvary HE not only defeated satan and his evil works but that HE purchased and sealed us for salvation. HE set us free from the evil bondage of sin and iniquities and infirmities [sickness] and delivered our healing to us by the stripes HE bore. Our problem is our reluctance to make a claim, by faith, to be resolved that we are GOD'S property and that GOD is Sovereign.

HEBREWS 11:6 BUT WITHOUT FAITH IT IS IMPOSSIBLE TO PLEASE HIM; FOR HE THAT COMETH TO GOD MUST BELIEVE THAT HE IS AND THAT HE IS A REWARDER OF THEM THAT DILIGENTLY SEEK HIM. JEWISH NEW TESTAMENT

We do not belong to satan and thus we can not serve an evil task master whose desire it is to steal, kill and destroy us and everything we hold precious.

It has been said that there are 39 root causes of illness, and it is public record in HIS SCRIPTURE that YESHUA received 39 stripes. Each strip was for us, for our healing. So why do we make claim to sickness? Why do so many allow the enemy of our soul to claim rule over our bodies? It is because of our failure to search for truth in HIS WORD, where HE lives and freely gives abundant life for the asking. A simple yet Holy way to salvation, still many choose to follow man's traditions and have failed to walk by faith, but rather to walk by sight, in lust of the eyes and pride of flesh.

EPHESIANS 6:11,12 PUT ON THE WHOLE ARMOR OF GOD, THAT YE MAY BE ABLE TO STAND AGAINST THE WILES OF THE DEVIL. 12. FOR WE WRESTLE NOT AGAINST FLESH AND BLOOD, BUT AGAINST PRINCIPALITIES, AGAINST POWERS, AGAINST THE RULERS OF DARKNESS OF THIS WORLD, AGAINST SPIRITUAL WICKEDNESS IN HIGH PLACES. JEWISH NEW TESTAMENT

The world screams an urgency for the people of GOD to pray and seek HIS Mercy and Grace, a work that only a supreme move of GOD can accomplish to enable us to have victory and healing and release from satans chains of bondage.

The expectant confidence of a believer is based on faith in the Character of GOD, who unlike man is full of mercy, truth and justice and expects those who call themselves by HIS NAME to be as HE is. Healing was always at the HEART of YESHUA'S ministry when HE lived on Earth and still today HIS promise of healing is alive and well.

ACTS 10:38 HOW GOD ANOINTED YESHUA THE MESSIAH WITH THE HOLY GHOST AND WITH POWER; WHO WENT ABOUT DOING GOOD, AND HEALING ALL THAT WERE

OPPRESSED OF THE DEVIL; FOR GOD WAS WITH HIM. JEWISH NEW TESTAMENT

If healing terminated at YESHUA'S death GOD forgot to tell the Apostles for they continued to heal with time. Healing was ushered into today and that is proven by GOD as HE sent back HIS HOLY SPIRIT as our teacher [mentor] after YESHUA went home to set at HIS RIGHT HAND on HIS throne of Glorious healing and abundant life.

If healing is not for today the BIBLE is a lie from start to finish but on the contrary, THE BIBLE is the only BOOK that is not a lie and the only BOOK that is alive and has survived numerous attempts by satan to destroy it time after time.

HEBREWS 4:12 FOR THE WORD OF GOD IS LIVING, AND POWERFUL AND SHARPER THAN ANY TWO EDGED SWORD, PIERCING EVEN TO THE DIVIDING ASUNDER OF SOUL AND SPIRIT, AND OF THE JOINTS AND MARROW, AND IS A DISCERNER OF THE THOUGHTS AND INTENTS OF THE HEART. JEWISH NEW TESTAMENT

GOD'S SCRIPTURE stands in judgment against the monarch of hell and his corrupt and immoral evil, but the majority of humanity is fixed in denial and rejection as they refuse to read or listen to HIS WORD. They do not realize HIS SUPREME POWER and the authority it offers to HIS CHILDREN.

Just as satan has attempted to destroy GOD'S WORD down through time, he attempts, every fleeting moment to destroy GOD'S people so we must determine to be wise and consume GOD'S WORD as a defense against this evil enemy.

ISAIAH 59:19 SO SHALL THEY FEAR THE NAME OF THE LORD FROM THE WEST AND HIS GLORY FROM THE RISING OF THE SUN.[EAST] WHEN THE ENEMY SHALL COME IN LIKE A FLOOD, THE SPIRIT OF THE LORD SHALL LIFT UP A STANDARD AGAINST HIM. JEWISH NEW TEST.

SCRIPTURE is like having unclaimed money in the bank. The difference is money [mammon] is temporal and the covenants from SCRIPTURES are never-ending. Our obstacles occur within our failure to make rightful claim. But our neglect to make claim is generally couched in the rejection of HIS WORD or in our unconcerned point of view to those assurances that were established at Calvary. Consequently our anxiety and doubt cause us to withdraw and we become terrified to step out in faith or perhaps we have been brain washed in vein traditions. Listened to the words of men who dwell and cherish vain fables in their much talk, when we need only to turn to SCRIPTURE to seek GOD and to listen as HE speaks reality and truth in love and mercy.

HEBREWS 11:26 ESTEEMING THE REPROACH OF CHRIST GREATER RICHES THAN THE TREASURES IN EGYPT FOR HE HAD RESPECT UNTO THE RECOMPENSE OF THE REWARD.

In ancient days Egypt was known as a pagan nation. Everywhere there were idolatrous people worshipping false images who were cruel and demanding of human sacrifice. Pagans who practiced sorcery and magic lived in fear of demons who were desperately corrupt. However today Egypt has lost her glory and stands as a monument to the dead as the large massive mummy tombs stand in lifeless memory of a self exalted nation. Symbolically Egypt is a type of slavery and bondage representative of the world today and we must resolve to remove our worldly shoes [symbolic] of vanity and pride and robe ourselves in righteousness so that we may be found worthy to enter before a HOLY AND JUST GOD our CREATOR, in praise and glory.

PSALMS 100:4 ENTER INTO HIS GATES WITH THANKSGIVING, AND INTO HIS COURTS WITH PRAISE; BE THANKFUL UNTO HIM AND BLESS HIS NAME.

As believers we should be a reflection of HIS WORD, a living breathing representation of joy, peace, and truth. When we begin to seek YESHUA we will begin to hunger for HIS WILL in our lives as we will slowly become that reflection to emulate HIM. Through HIS WORD we can conquer the devil in our life with our testimony and walking by faith will appear as natural as a bird in flight.

We will celebrate GOD'S STANDARD of light when the prince of darkness comes toward us and dynamically announce our completeness in YESHUA. Even if we are disfigured or in a wheel chair we can be triumphant and illustrate HIS LOVE. Being convinced that our circumstance is temporary. Our everlastingness has been obtained where we will be flawless and consummated in HEAVEN. It is only a matter of transitory passing from this life to be with THE LORD in Glory. Our willingness to commit to HIS WILL in this life is the key to answered petitions and victorious living through HIM.

GOD alone is the healer of our soul. What ever our lot, whether it be joy, peace, and righteousness or sin, sickness, and disease, etc., that presents itself in our body is seated in our soul, in our HEART. The two powers that we are bound by are in direct contrast to one another, we can not serve both. However our motivation is derived from the ONE we embrace to promote. GOD'S natural course is health and well being and GOD'S enemy satan's, is disease and death.

43

KILLER - ATTITUDE

ATTITUDE is a Spirit, a decided, determined and sometimes even sought after disposition that will reflect the god of self or the GOD of life.

Our attitude always determines the effect of any decision on our mind, heart, thought and emotion. We come under divine scrutiny and GOD'S ear is always open to those who are inwardly upright and sometimes even to the wicked. G O D ' S government is characterized by Holiness, HIS thoughts are moral to the highest degree and the cleansing of sin is essential for our salvation.

Consider the hard HEART caused by refusing to obey GOD. It stops up blood veins, causes HEART attacks, makes breathing erratic, makes the energy level low and thus we are unable to function as we should and many die from the 'hard HEART'. The Hard HEART turned to stone, has stopped the life line of blood and cut off existence, for life is in the blood.

By refusing GOD'S redemption we condemn ourselves but by allowing HIM to enter our HEART and confessing our sin, we gain new life, a new HEART.

EZK. 36:26 AND I WILL GIVE YOU A NEW HEART AND PUT A NEW SPIRIT WITHIN YOU; I WILL REMOVE THE HEART OF STONE FROM YOUR BODY AND GIVE YOU A HEART OF FLESH; :27 I WILL PUT MY SPIRIT INTO YOU. THUS I WILL CAUSE YOU TO FOLLOW MY LAWS AND FAITHFULLY TO OBSERVE MY RULES. JEWISH TANAKH

When we repent from our HEART, we realize how unfit we are and are humbled before GOD. HE promises to restore us by HIS GRACE and as unfit as we are, GOD meets us at the point of our need with HIS MERCY to cleanse us from the pollution of sin. Under HIS submission HE purifies our conscience and takes away our sense of guilt.

The HEART of stone, is insensible and inapt to receive divine impressions and therefore unable to return devout affections. But GOD will replace "it" with a soft and tender HEART of flesh that has spiritual senses exercised, complying in everything with HIS DIVINE LOVE. We will have been dipped in the Jordan of HIS precious and perfect Blood to come up washed as white as snow, with a new HEART, a new disposition and a new mind that will be clear to think good thoughts.

HEBREWS 4:7b TODAY IF YE WILL HEAR HIS VOICE, HARDEN NOT YOUR HEARTS. JEWISH NEW TESTAMENT

GOD'S WORD calls forth an inevitable reaction; men either respond in obedience to HIS CALL or stubbornly reject it. Rejection, which must be avoided, is the deceitfulness of sin, through which men's HEARTS are hardened against GOD and causes consequent unbelief that leads men to fall away or apostatize and become seduced to abandonment of response to GOD altogether.

Our life lies in the PRECIOUS BLOOD OF YESHUA, not the blood of man or beast. As the end of YESHUA'S walk on earth drew near, HE gathered HIS Disciples around HIMSELF in the upper room hoping to help them understand HIS MISSION as well as HIS DEATH as HE related the meaning of the PESACH [PASSOVER] in:

LUKE 22:17 THEN, TAKING A CUP OF WINE, HE MADE THE B'RAKHAH [BLESSING] AND SAID, "TAKE THIS AND SHARE IT AMONG YOURSELVES. :18 FOR I TELL YOU THAT FROM NOW ON, I WILL NOT DRINK THE 'FRUIT OF THE VINE' UNTIL THE KINGDOM OF GOD COMES." "19 ALSO, TAKING A PIECE OF MATZAH [UNLEAVENED BREAD-signifies life without sin] HE MADE THE B'RAKHAH [BLESSING], BROKE IT, GAVE IT TO THEM AND SAID, "THIS IS MY BODY, WHICH IS BEING GIVEN FOR YOU; DO THIS IN MEMORY OF ME" :20 HE DID THE SAME WITH THE CUP AFTER THE MEAL, SAYING, "THIS CUP IS THE NEW COVENANT, RATIFIED BY MY BLOOD, WHICH IS BEING POURED OUT FOR YOU." JEWISH NEW TESTAMENT

ROMANS 5:8 BUT GOD DEMONSTRATES HIS OWN LOVE FOR US IN THAT THE MESSIAH [CHRIST] DIED ON OUR BEHALF WHILE WE WERE STILL SINNERS. :9 THEREFORE, SINCE WE HAVE NOW COME TO BE CONSIDERED RIGHTEOUS BY MEANS OF HIS BLOODY SACRIFICIAL DEATH, HOW MUCH MORE WILL WE BE DELIVERED THROUGH HIM FROM THE ANGER OF GOD'S JUDGMENT. JEWISH NEW TESTAMENT

EPHESIANS 1:7 IN UNION WITH HIM, THROUGH THE SHEDDING OF HIS BLOOD, WE ARE SET FREE, OUR SINS ARE FORGIVEN; THIS ACCORDS WITH THE WEALTH OF THE GRACE :8 HE HAS LAVISHED ON US. IN ALL HIS WISDOM AND INSIGHT. JEWISH NEW TESTAMENT

HEBREWS 9:22 IN FACT, ACCORDING TO THE TORAH [LAW], ALMOST EVERYTHING IS PURIFIED WITH BLOOD;

INDEED, WITHOUT THE SHEDDING OF BLOOD THERE IS
NO FORGIVENESS OF SINS.
JEWISH NEW TESTAMENT

We are saved and cleansed by the Blood of YESHUA THE
MESSIAH, and when we choose to follow HIM, it is HIS BLOOD
that will flow in our veins because we are enjoined and become a
part of HIS family. HIS BLOOD is perfect, having no aliens of sin,
no trace of disease.

HEBREWS 9:11 BUT WHEN THE MESSIAH [JESUS] APPEARED
AS COHEN GADOL [HIGH PRIEST] OF THE GOOD THINGS
THAT ARE HAPPENING ALREADY, THEN, THROUGH THE
GREATER AND MORE PERFECT TENT WHICH IS NOT
MAN-MADE :12 HE ENTERED THE HOLIEST PLACE ONCE
AND FOR ALL. :13 AND HE ENTERED NOT BY MEANS OF
BLOOD OF GOATS AND CALVES, BUT BY MEANS OF HIS
OWN BLOOD, THUS SETTING PEOPLE FREE FOREVER. :13
FOR IF SPRINKLING CEREMONIALLY UNCLEAN PERSONS
WITH BLOOD OF GOATS AND BULLS AND THE ASHES OF
A HEIFER RESTORES THEIR OUTWARD PURITY; :14 THEN
HOW MUCH MORE THE BLOOD OF THE MESSIAH, WHO,
THROUGH THE ETERNAL SPIRIT, OFFERED HIMSELF
TO GOD AS A SACRIFICE WITHOUT BLEMISH, WILL
PURIFY OUR CONSCIENCE FROM WORKS THAT LEAD TO
DEATH, SO THAT WE CAN SERVE THE LIVING GOD. :15
IT IS BECAUSE OF THIS DEATH THAT HE IS MEDIATOR
OF A NEW COVENANT [OR WILL]. BECAUSE A DEATH
HAS OCCURRED WHICH SETS PEOPLE FREE FROM THE
TRANSGRESSIONS COMMITTED UNDER THE FIRST
COVENANT, THOSE WHO HAVE BEEN CALLED MAY
RECEIVE THE PROMISED ETERNAL INHERITANCE.
JEWISH NEW TESTAMENT

We become like HIM when we learn to love others, as HE loves us, forgive others as HE has forgiven us, do for others as HE does for us even to the endth degree of our life.

The difference lies in our choice of who we serve.

COLOSSIANS 1:21 IN OTHER WORDS, YOU, WHO AT ONE TIME WERE SEPARATED FROM GOD AND HAD A HOSTILE ATTITUDE TOWARDS HIM BECAUSE OF YOUR WICKED DEEDS, :22 HE HAS NOW RECONCILED IN THE SON'S PHYSICAL BODY THROUGH HIS DEATH; IN ORDER TO PRESENT YOU HOLY AND WITHOUT DEFECT OR REPROACH BEFORE HIMSELF :23 PROVIDED, OF COURSE, THAT YOU CONTINUE IN YOUR TRUSTING, GROUNDED AND STEADY, AND DON'T LET YOURSELVES BE MOVED AWAY FROM THE HOPE OFFERED IN THE GOOD NEWS YOU HEARD. JEWISH NEW TESTAMENT

LITTLE BATTLE SHIPS

An attitude of anger and bitterness will record in the HEART and will begin or add severe and irrefutable damage making the flow of Blood all but impossible after a while. This attitude will send messages of pain and stress out to the 'LITTLE SHIPS' [corpuscles] that maintain our healthy flow of blood.

HEBREWS 12:14 KEEP PURSUING SHALOM [PEACE] WITH EVERYONE AND THE HOLINESS WITHOUT WHICH NO ONE WILL SEE THE LORD. :15 SEE TO IT THAT NO ONE MISSES OUT ON, GOD'S GRACE, THAT NO ROOT OF BITTERNESS SPRINGING UP CAUSES TROUBLE AND THUS CONTAMINATES MANY AND, :16 AND THAT NO ONE IS SEXUALLY IMMORAL, OR GODLESS LIKE ESAV [ESAU] WHO IN EXCHANGE FOR A SINGLE MEAL GAVE UP HIS RIGHTS AS THE FIRSTBORN :17 FOR YOU KNOW THAT AFTERWARDS, WHEN HE WANTED TO OBTAIN HIS FATHER'S BLESSING, HE WAS REJECTED; INDEED, EVEN

THOUGH HE SOUGHT IT WITH TEARS, HIS CHANGE OF
HEART WAS TO NO AVAIL. JEWISH NEW TESTAMENT

If we are not careful to keep check on our attitude, we will
be subjected to the little bad attitude attacks and each assault of
hostility or festering anger releases noxious little bombs to those
'little ships', even when numerous bombs hit a large ship it will
ultimately destroy it, and if the noxious little bomb attacks of
anger, bitterness, jealousy, selfishness, etc. are admitted to travel
in our veins and carry through to strike the 'little ships' they will
in due time destroy us. The little bombs will continue to go on to
the next and the next and the next until our veins become callused
and hard due to the battle going on within.

The messages of indifference to GOD'S WILL are full of
destructive forces. If left unchecked they will conquer and
vanquish the fragile 'little ships' and as the "sick ships" yield to
disease and disappear, the robust "ships" are left to over load under
attack. Eventually all the 'little corpuscle ships' are in torment and
too feeble to encounter any more enemies, our immune system
is doomed. Our 'little ships', veins and body has given up and we
have become to weak, to sick and to diseased. The immune system
has failed and thrown open doors for permanent impairment or
possible death.

The destructive forces have grown and festered until all the
'little corpuscle ships' in the Blood Stream are defeated. The shores
[outer walls of veins] begin to be attack and disease moves to the
out side of the body in the form of sores, cancer, diabetes, arthritis,
new phenomena, aids, etc. satan and his armored division of evil
spirits have affirmed their presence in the system and taken over
GOD'S Creative Image and are masterminding the conclusive
attack of death. The ocean of our life has become discouraging
and detached in darkness. Dare we give our soul up to the enemy
never to understand the healing victory of YESHUA? Dare we
allow the enemy to blind us and take us into his dirty, firey, hellish

kingdom? Dare we wallow in our own self pity, controlled by our sickness? Do we accept defeat from the enemy or do we look up and claim the LIGHT?

If we would [not could] grab hold of the hem of YESHUA'S Robe, just as the lady with the issue of blood did and make claim [believe] in THE NAME OF YESHUA for HIS DIVINE Healing Power that HE left to us at Calvary, we could claim victory and free ourselves of the bondage of torment the monarch of hell cast over our lives because we did not realize our authority in YESHUA. Dare we be so bold as to claim our rights stolen by the devil?

LUKE 8:43,44 AND A WOMAN HAVING AS ISSUE OF BLOOD [HEMORRHAGE]OF TWELVE YEARS, WHICH HAD SPENT ALL HER LIVING UPON PHYSICIANS, NEITHER COULD BE HEALED OF ANY. 44. CAME BEHIND HIM AND TOUCHED THE BORDER OF HIS GARMENT; AND IMMEDIATELY HER ISSUE OF BLOOD STANCHED.

JEWISH NEW TESTAMENT

This woman's hemorrhage refused to yield to doctors and inasmuch as her affliction made her religiously unclean she was frightened to encounter YESHUA in the open. Her faith was sufficient to have no doubt that HE was the DIVINE HEALER and if she could but touch even the hem of HIS garment, she had faith [attitude] that she would be healed and she was right, for as she struggled to brush against the hem of HIS robe through the pushing and pulling of the crowd, she felt her body be restored and she was made whole instantly. YESHUA'S reason to call her out was to restore her self respect by making public her relationship with HIMSELF as the HEALER, freeing her and all who knew her from suspicion of superstition.

Those of us who declare we 'cannot' are obligated by the cords of our sin and our attitude is isolated in callousness as our condition is sealed by our words of "cannot" which deem our state of being as unrelenting, oppressive and self-inflicted.

DARE WE LOOK TO YESHUA?! What admirable throne do we pride ourselves with as we bury our kisser in the pillow[symbolic] of self pity, weeping for ourselves? Dare we gain victory by simply turning to YESHUA IN REPENTANCE, giving to HIM our stubborn will and HEART? For only HE has the authority and the longing to reinstate all that the canker worm has destroyed and HE alone finds pleasure in giving us abundant life in return for obedience. HE will restore that impenetrable, unrelenting HEART and deposit a new HEART that will issue uncontaminated vigor. But only for those who BELIEVE!

EZK. 36:26 A NEW HEART ALSO WILL I GIVE YOU, AND A NEW SPIRIT WILL I PUT WITHIN YOU; AND I WILL TAKE AWAY THE STONY HEART OUT OF YOUR FLESH, AND I WILL GIVE YOU AN HEART OF FLESH.

GOD will replace the 'little corpuscle ships' and the shorelines [veins] eaten by sin and disease. HE will cleanse the foul matter and rottenness without hesitation that the devil has put into position on top of the walking anesthetized man. HE will style our lives and cover us with righteous robes, white as snow that prepare us to go before HIS FATHER who will adopt us into HIS FAMILY; the ROYAL FAMILY OF GOD.

EZK. 18:30b REPENT AND TURN YOURSELVES FROM ALL YOUR TRANSGRESSION; SO INIQUITY SHALL NOT BE YOUR RUIN.

JEWISH NEW TESTAMENT

CHOOSE THIS DAY WHO YOU WILL SERVE.

MATTHEW 6:24 NO ONE CAN BE SLAVE TO TWO MASTERS; FOR HE WILL EITHER HATE THE FIRST AND LOVE THE SECOND, OR SCORN THE SECOND AND BE LOYAL TO THE FIRST. YOU CAN'T BE A SLAVE TO BOTH GOD AND MONEY. JEWISH NEW TESTAMENT

The New HEART and New MIND are synonymous with the blessings of THE HOLY SPIRIT and can only be assumed from GOD. It is a supernatural gift to be cherished, inhaled and adored. It is not to be rationalized as a simple inspiration of man.

The questions and answers of this world reflect only hopelessness and despair of our current situation and there's no answer but YESHUA. GOD urges us in HIS WORD time and time again, "LET NOT YOUR HEART BE HARDENED".

PROVERBS 29:1 ONE OFT REPROVED MAY BECOME STIFF NECKED, BUT HE WILL BE SUDDENLY BROKEN BEYOND REPAIR.

JEWISH TANAKH

Head strong wills are so masterful that if GOD should leave us wholly to the wilderness of our unruly nature, to take our own course, we would soon run ourselves upon our own ruin.

ISAIAH 3:8b BECAUSE THEIR TONGUE AND THEIR DOINGS ARE AGAINST THE LORD, TO PROVOKE THE EYES OF HIS GLORY. 9. THE SHOP OF THEIR COUNTENANCE DOTH WITNESS AGAINST THEM, AND THEY DECLARE THEIR SIN LIKE SODOM; THEY HIDE IT NOT. WOE UNTO THEIR SOUL! FOR THEY HAVE REWARDED EVIL UNTO THEMSELVES. JEWISH NEW TESTAMENT

The skeptic may have a fling in his own self confidence but in the end he will be left stranded in the wasteland he has produced. He has damned his eternity by the impenetrable attitude of his HEART.

GOD'S attribute of Holiness cannot be modified or changed. HIS justice is sure and as we rebel and brace our neck, it shackles our HEART, instantly our ears become clogged to keep us from aspiring towards GOD'S WORDS, we have invited GOD'S judgment. Every beating pulse of one who sins is rebellion against a GOD of love WHO mounts HIS relentless wrath through HIS sharpened WORD where HIS justice is found and directed to the one who sins and denies HIS Grace and mercy. The conduct of the transgressor will cast off GOD'S protection, blessings and glory.

PROVERBS 21:29 A WICKED MAN HARDENETH HIS FACE; BUT AS FOR THE UPRIGHT HE DIRECTETH HIS WAY.

A hardened face, without shame or blushing for iniquity is a fearful manifestation of a hardened HEART and is determined to do wickedness. The HEART is repulsive and the very idea of the grace of GOD is an object of scorn and contempt. He covers himself with garments of wickedness, shame, misery, disease and dishonor as he walks as a dead man in his own self-righteousness, dirty rags.

Evil is the nature of the wicked HEART and is fully set to be corrupt and depraved. The appetite craves evil and evil has become the main delight. The vessels of an evil person are full of sin and therefore full of wrath, disease and death. GOD responds to sin with rewards of punishment for all who practice dominate disregard for HIS LAW.

Fidelity unto GOD leads to the cross and emphasizes repentance from the HEART. The desire to change becomes a reality as we move into divine submission to our Creator GOD, WHO alone judges the HEART and will search and expose any remaining wickedness as well as lead us in the way of eternal life.

PSALMS 139:23 'SEARCH ME O GOD AND KNOW MY HEART; TRY ME AND KNOW MY THOUGHTS; 24. SEE IF THERE BE ANY WICKED WAY IN ME AND LEAD ME IN THE WAY EVERLASTING.

The world has only contempt for those who profess to be GOD'S people, whose lives are inconsistent with their profession while even the unbeliever will respect those who diligently walk the walk and talk the talk.

SPIRIT OF EVIL IS KILLER OF OUR HEART

Our HEARTS are callused by means of the decisions we give rise to in our own unrestricted will and GOD loves the unassuming, meek humble person but despises the prideful and self righteous. There is a divine relationship between the HEART and health and GOD'S unique standard is predetermined for each individual at birth. HE provides the air for breathing, a tongue and dialect for communication. HE has sovereignty over all creation and created each person distinctive in HIS Image and for HIS pleasure. But the man of flesh sought a self focused trail to follow therefore made himself subject to all evil, he has no defense for battle for the war is not by flesh but by spirits of the vilest evil.

EPHESIANS 6:10 FINALLY, GROW POWERFUL IN UNION WITH THE LORD, IN UNION WITH HIS MIGHTY STRENGTH! :11 USE ALL THE ARMOR AND WEAPONRY THAT GOD PROVIDES, SO THAT YOU WILL BE ABLE TO STAND AGAINST THE DECEPTIVE TACTICS OF

THE ADVERSARY. :12 FOR <u>WE ARE NOT STRUGGLING</u> <u>AGAINST HUMAN BEINGS, BUT AGAINST THE RULERS,</u> <u>AUTHORITIES AND COSMIC POWERS GOVERNING THIS</u> <u>DARKNESS, AGAINST THE SPIRITUAL FORCES OF EVIL IN</u> <u>THE HEAVENLY REALM</u>. JEWISH NEW TESTAMENT

REVELATION 16:14 THEY ARE <u>MIRACLE-WORKING</u> <u>DEMONIC SPIRITS</u> WHICH GO OUT TO THE KINGS OF THE WHOLE INHABITED WORLD TO ASSEMBLE THEM FOR THE WAR OF THE GREAT DAY OF ADONAI-TZVA'OT. {THE LORD, JEHOVAH OF HOSTS} JEWISH NEW TESTAMENT

Demon spirits are foul, demonic, loathsome, and offensive. If we are not in GOD'S WILL and seeking HIS WAY in obedience, and satan does not see GOD as our protector and shield , man is only flesh and the devil prepares to devour him. Only under GOD'S guardianship does satan see YESHUA'S BLOOD and this DIVINE BLOOD is the exclusive pure and just covering that causes satan to shrivel and recoil, for. satan can not make an entrance by way of that Precious Blood and thus the prince of darkness trembles and is conquered in the magnificent light of YESHUA.

In our unspiritual and carnal individualism we fear man. We have a tendency to withdraw from disapproval and obligation and rationalize around the CROSS to find excuses for abnormal perverted feelings that we wish to indulge. Those things we want to explore and places we yearn to go take priority. We are enamored with mother earth and the terrestrial sphere {astrology} and to love the world is enmity with GOD.

However even for the sinner, after a while the weight of transgression cultivates and permeates a full to overflowing dimension of guiltiness. Judgment becomes depressingly burdensome and GOD'S justice stands as a eyewitness face-to-face with us. GOD'S wrath is overwhelming. If we are still breathing, even now we can convert our viewpoint to reach for

GOD from within and escape the wickedness of satan with our HEART to obtain eternal life..

DEUTERONOMY 32:39 SEE NOW, THAT I, EVEN I, AM HE, AND THERE IS NO GOD WITH ME, I KILL, AND I MAKE ALIVE; I WOUND, AND I HEAL; NEITHER IS THERE ANY THAT CAN DELIVER OUT OF MY HAND.

Only in YESHUA'S SPIRIT can we become one who 'HOPETH ALL THINGS, ENDURETH ALL THINGS' but when GOD is with us there are no demons or man that can convert or claim us.

GOD'S purpose is truth and goodness and it's practice is safety. Only through YESHUA, by GOD'S forgiveness and grace can sin and disease lose their challenge to our minds [consciousness]. As darkness gives way to light thus sin gives way to SALVATION. The sinner when touched by truth becomes convinced, and only then is he willing to allow GOD to become his master molder. For GOD reproves any darkness from HIS WORD, which mirrors all our faults.

Illness, disease and stress is often the exterior manifestation of a deeply buried and in all likelihood dangerous battle going on inside. Anger, jealousy and bitterness, hate, etc., are divinely recorded in the blood vessels, the heart, intestines, muscles, nervous system, eyes, brain and body. Furthermore when we experience these emotions, and make a decision to engage and celebrate them, they insist on being reported as deficients in our system. Sickness and impairment will initiate and commence to manifest and to deliberately eat away at our soundness of mind and body. They will linger and loiter and continue to sponsor their repulsive properties and increase as long as we reject GOD and spurn forgiveness. We remain guilty and guiltiness is a killer. Our only immunity and freedom comes through the Precious Blood of YESHUA and it is accessible, convenient and profitable for our election.

JAMES 2:10 FOR A PERSON WHO KEEPS THE WHOLE TORAH [LAW], YET STUMBLES AT ONE POINT, HAS BECOME GUILTY OF BREAKING THEM ALL. :11 FOR THE ONE WHO SAID, "DON'T COMMIT ADULTERY," ALSO SAID, "DON'T MURDER." NOW IF YOU DON'T COMMIT ADULTERY BUT DO MURDER, YOU HAVE BECOME A TRANSGRESSOR OF THE TORAH. :12 KEEP SPEAKING AND ACTING LIKE PEOPLE WHO WILL BE JUDGED BY A TORAH [LAW] WHICH GIVES FREEDOM. :13 FOR JUDGMENT WILL BE WITHOUT MERCY TOWARD ONE WHO DOESN'T SHOW MERCY; BUT MERCY WINS OUT OVER JUDGMENT. JEWISH NEW TESTAMENT

A defiant and brazen perspective and a callused HEART will seize a disposition and progress to make a person as good as unreachable. Because when a HEART grows stony against GOD, it is about to be on the rocks.

Dare we see that if we confess...HE will forgive? There is no reason to pack around the ball and chain of satan's bondage. The simplicity of seeking GOD is somehow baffling to the hard HEARTED but locking the closeted chamber of sin gives authorization to an oppressive and dark future.

The world's worst and loneliest prison is the HEART and when iniquity is locked within it empties life of all the good things. Our only assurance is in The LORD and when sins are confessed a heavy burden is lifted right off the HEART. We can rest assured that honest confession receives forgiveness. Freedom-giving forgiveness. -

As one man said, "Almost anything in the world can be bought for money - except the warm impulses of the human HEART. They have to be given. And they are priceless in their power to purchase happiness for two people, the recipient and the giver."

Guilt is another evil spirit that is a health robber. Many times it is sin unconfessed, seated deep in the unconscious and by evil design allowed to block healing. It gives birth to a dungeon that far eclipses Alcatraz's horror and is hidden in the solitary confinement to reveal how a person feels when chained by unconfessed sin and guilt. As the conscience eats at the HEART day after day about the miserable guiltiness packaged with in the invisible confines and bars of the prison we have personally formed, it will create walls of stress that confirm HEART disease as well as dishonor and shame.

True guilt is the deep conviction of sin and the result of the HOLY SPIRIT speaking through a tender conscience.. The moral elements of sin constitute a hell of themselves, apart from the material fire. The fruit of sin in time, when arrived to full and finished maturity, is just the fruit of sin through eternity. It is merely the sinner reaping what he has sown and it must be confessed to GOD to be conquered.

1 JOHN 1:8 IF WE CLAIM NOT TO HAVE SIN, WE ARE DECEIVING OURSELVES, AND THE TRUTH IS NOT IN US. :9 IF WE ACKNOWLEDGE OUR SINS, THEN, SINCE HE IS TRUSTWORTHY AND JUST, HE WILL FORGIVE THEM AND PURIFY US FROM ALL WRONG DOING. JEWISH NEW TESTAMENT

WISDOM has solemnly warned the rebellious scorner through out GOD'S WORD that we must confront and confess sin through HIS Grace, we must lay it down and go past it. Acknowledge it to GOD and seek HIS forgiveness to continue on to newness of life. That is the seed cast into the ground of an honest and good HEART, a HEART prepared for GOD.

By forgiving others, we will open the door for our own forgiveness from the HEAVENLY FATHER, to enter our HEART and make good health conceivable. Forgiveness can not be earned and it not optional, it is a righteousness offered by GOD as a gift bestowed, not a right to be claimed.

In contrast , 'EVIL COMMUNICATIONS CORRUPT GOOD MANNERS'. If we endure faithful and remember that every step on satan's ground deprives us of the security of the promises of GOD, our dealings will be blessed as well as our coming and going. However, when we refuse to deal with sin in a constructive manner it will begin to fester and poison the HEART. It becomes an open wound of self infliction as satan sets out for slaughter, unconsciously we begin seeking accidents, misery, torment and suffering. Sin is a symptom of the self destructive force on the rampage.

ROMANS 4:7 BLESSED ARE THEY WHOSE TRANSGRESSIONS ARE FORGIVEN AND WHOSE SINS ARE COVERED.

SPIRIT OF PRIDE

A spirit of pride always exalts its position and success to peacock with conceit. Example: As pride enters a room, dressed in the most expensive, luxurious and frilly garment, the prideful inter-person is enamored with human praise and a fondness to be noticed. It loves supremacy and glories in attention of self in passing or conversation and is exalted when there is a free time of speaking or praying to indulge in intellectual hypocrisy. Unaware that beauty is only skin deep and fashion is temporary but ugliness goes all the way to the bone and stems from the HEART. It seems no matter how shallow beauty and fashion are the prideful, arrogant soul wants it. What pride does not realize is that GOD places no premium on cheekbones, eyes, curves, dress or fashion but HE is a stickler for the inner beauty that comes from a clean, pure and humble HEART.

'VILE AVARICE AND PRIDE, FROM HEAVEN ACCURST)

IN ALL ARE ILL, BUT IN A CHURCH-MAN WORST.

BY: SIR WILLIAM ALEXANDER, EARL OF STIRLING
"DOOMSDAY"

Pride is insidious. It will cause one to be impatient and ambitious for it invades every facet of a person's life for contamination and destruction.. As we become angered when another does not move out of our way or understand our reasoning, it is the enemy that has employed our system for the purpose of belittling or even destroying another. Whether we call it nervousness or holy indignation it is a touchy, sensitive spirit that resents and retaliates when disapproved of or contradicted.

Our pride will make us self willed, stubborn, and unteachable. Our behavior will be arrogant, we will prance about in full blown conceit to eventually become our thoughts.

In the 1800's George Mueller, a mighty prayer warrior when ask what his secret was, he responded,

"THERE WAS A DAY WHEN I DIED; DIED TO GEORGE MUELLER, HIS OPINIONS, PREFERENCES, TASTES, AND WILL; DIED TO THE WORLD, ITS APPROVAL OR CENSURE; DIED TO THE APPROVAL OR BLAME OF MY BRETHREN AND FRIENDS; AND SINCE THEN I HAVE STUDIED ONLY TO SHOW MYSELF APPROVED UNTO GOD."

When pride dies, greatness begins. YESHUA taught that when HE said;

MATTHEW 23:12 FOR WHOEVER PROMOTES HIMSELF WILL BE HUMBLED, AND WHOEVER HUMBLES HIMSELF WILL BE PROMOTED.

JEWISH NEW TESTAMENT.

Pride makes our spirit argumentative, harsh, sarcastic, unyielding, headstrong and commanding, we develop a critical disposition and find fault with the imperfections of others. We simply refuse to be overlooked or ignored. It is ego fed and with each feast it bloats, gloats and then pops.

SHAKESPEARE ONCE SAID,"HE THAT IS PROUD EATS UP HIMSELF."

But there is a superhighway out of this grave adversity that we have fabricated in our driving enterprise to become important. The way down from the mountain of pride is through the valley of humiliation and it is deep and rugged, nevertheless there is more to gain on the journey down than was acquired on the uppity expedition. A peaceable and remorseful consciousness will be rewarded and respected and the compensation is eternal life. But an exalted disrespectful and doubtful man, full of his own thoughts is eaten up with cancerous self superiority and his end will be in the abyss.

PROVERBS 8:13 THE FEAR OF THE LORD IS TO HATE EVIL; PRIDE, AND ARROGANCE, AND THE EVIL WAY, AND THE PERVERSE MOUTH, DO I HATE.

Pride is a sin that GOD finds abominable for it is a poisonous weed. When it is cultivated and watered it will take root in the HEART. As growth matures it chokes out goodness and righteousness and replaces them with hardened and rotten decay that ultimately destroys the inner system. Consequently, it has prepared the HEART for failures and diseases.

Like unto a vine that grows out of the ground and wraps around a mature tree, as it matures it gets stronger and larger. Eventually it will be so strong and large that the lovely tree grows weak and slowly dies. It's destruction could have been stopped by cutting away the root but it wasn't and now the tree has been slowly choked to death. Thus does sin slowly wrap itself around our veins and HEART to smother life for sin in the heart creates native soil for the sin nature.

PROVERBS 11:2 WHEN PRIDE COMETH, THEN COMETH SHAME

PROVERBS 16:18 PRIDE GOETH BEFORE DESTRUCTION & AN HAUGHTY SPIRIT BEFORE A FALL

Let us examine secret faults from the HEART source. Do we place a subtle confidence in gifts, attainments and privileges? God hates pride and vows to bring it down because of HIS justice and by HIS judgment. Often GOD will smite the object of those things we most cherish, the high thoughts or items that set highest in our HEART. That makes us proud, HE will use those 'things' to bring us down. It is the state of the HEART that prepares man to fall, for what is our pride is our danger.

Thomas Adam declared, "PRIDE THRUST NEBUCHADNEZZAR OUT OF MEN'S SOCIETY, SAUL OUT OF HIS KINGDOM, ADAM OUT OF PARADISE, HAMAN OUT OF COURT, AND lucifer OUT OF HEAVEN."

AUGUSTINE NAMED PRIDE AS THE GREATEST OF ALL SINS, POINTING OUT THAT WHEN MAN IS PROUD HE EXALTS HIMSELF AND DISPLEASES GOD.

DEFOR SPOKE OF PRIDE AS THE FIRST PIER AND PRESIDENT OF HELL.

ALEXANDER POPE SAID THAT PRIDE WAS THE NEVER FAILING VICE OF FOOLS.

CS LEWIS CALLS PRIDE THE COMPLETE anti-god STATE OF MIND.

WEBSTER DEFINES PRIDE AS A QUALITY OR STATE OF BEING PROUD; AS INORDINATE SELF ESTEEM; CONCEIT.

Righteous piety {pride} is essentially concerned with the ethical, not the externals. It is synonymous with self respect and personal dignity in a good sense but mismanaged pride is synonymous with self esteem, self importance, arrogance and similar vices.

Pride is hated by GOD and it generates from an evil HEART to defile man, pictured here is one of the perilous times of the last days in

2 TIM. 3:1-5 MOREOVER, UNDERSTAND THIS: IN THE ACHARIT-HAYAMIM {LAST DAYS} WILL COME TRYING TIMES. :2 PEOPLE WILL BE SELF-LOVING, MONEY-LOVING, PROUD, ARROGANT, INSULTING, DISOBEDIENT TO PARENTS, UNGRATEFUL, UNHOLY, :3 HEARTLESS, UNAPPEASABLE, SLANDEROUS, UNCONTROLLED, BRUTAL, HATEFUL OF GOOD, :4 TRAITOROUS, HEADSTRONG, SWOLLEN WITH CONCEIT, LOVING PLEASURE RATHER THAN GOD, :5 AS THEY RETAIN THE OUTER FORM OF RELIGION BUT DENY ITS POWER. JEWISH NEW TEST.

It was pride that caused the first sin of murder on earth between brothers and is the root of all sin. It was the cause of satan's fall from Heaven and it can keep us from entering into "the" Heaven if we are not willing to put down our worldly possessions and seek GOD. It will keep us too proud to be humble or confess our sin. It will prevent one from saying I'm sorry to some one we have wronged and it always results in tragedy if left unchecked.

The egotism of pride can cause us to live beyond our means as we strive to 'keep up with the Jones' and it will motive us do things to make an impression on others but when the outgo exceeds the income the upkeep will be the downfall. The ambition to do well is far better than the ambition to be well to do.

PROVERBS 13:10 PRIDE CAUSES CONTENTION

PSALMS 10:4 PRIDE LEADS TO REBELLION

32 JOHN 9,10 PRIDE CAUSES A RULE OR RUIN ATTITUDE;

1 TIM. 3:6; PROVERBS 16:18;1 COR. 10:12 PRIDE LEADS TO APOSTASY.

When we faithfully seek GOD, HE will strip the unholy pride and deliver us from the darkness of mental and physical pain, weariness of doubt and discord to ransom our soul by HIS light of wholeness and liveliness of victory and transplant a new and vivacious HEART that will energize the whole system.

1 PETER 2:9 THAT YE SHOULD SHOW THE PRAISES OF HIM WHO HATH CALLED YOU OUT OF DARKNESS INTO HIS MARVELOUS LIGHT.

Far to often HE calls us out of darkness, forgives our sin, removes our sickness, and absent mindedly we forget or refuse to be thankful by seeking HIS WORD. . We forgot to give HIM thanks and praise for HIS gifts and become discouraged. The enemy is lurking to find that open door of return to usher us right back into our old life as usual, as if nothing had happened and as satan re-enters he brings all of the same ailments and idolatries coupled with more doubt than before. Only this time he brings more of his demon associates who are more vile, to dwell once more in our 'temple..

Thus friends look down in disbelief of how we have scorned and disappointed them after all the hard work. Forgetting that some perhaps also came from that same pit yet do not remember the struggle to break the heavy chains of death that satan wraps one with.

We must all remember what YESHUA said to all the people as they crowded around the woman, whose HEARTS were set to stone the maiden, but HE challenged all who stood before HIM in their pride and self righteousness. HE said

"HE WHO IS WITHOUT SIN THROW THE FIRST STONE"

After they had gone HE told the woman

"GO AND SIN NO MORE"

HIS statement was an important and essential WORD that reflected HIS HEART and is beneficial for each of us in this time. If we will seek HIM and put away our own self importance, we will be blessed with good health and wisdom. HE will renew our HEART each morning and give us HIS pure and righteous WISDOM that will manage our time every day, if we but ask. HE is a THE HEAVENLY FATHER and a good FATHER that desires above all else our obedience for which HE returns abundant life. The conscientiousness that our goings are of the LORD will give energy to our faith and our HEART will mend and be confident of GOD as our great physician.

PSALMS 51:9 PURGE ME WITH HYSSOP TILL I AM PURE; WASH ME TILL I AM WHITER THAN SNOW. :10 LET ME HEAR TIDINGS OF JOY AND GLADNESS; LET THE BONES YOU HAVE CRUSHED EXULT. :11 HIDE YOUR FACE FROM MY SINS; BLOT OUT ALL MYINIQUITIES. :12 FASHION A PURE HEART FOR ME, O GOD; CREATE IN ME A STEADFAST SPIRIT. :13 DO NOT CAST ME OUT OF YOUR PRESENCE, OR TAKE YOUR HOLY SPIRIT AWAY FROM ME. LET ME AGAIN REJOICE IN YOUR HELP; LET A VIGOROUS SPIRIT SUSTAIN ME. :15 I WILL TEACH TRANSGRESSORS YOUR WAYS, THAT SINNERS MAY RETURN TO YOU. JEWISH TANAKH

Where there is grace in the HEART there is healing in the tongue. We ourselves owe everything to GOD'S free grace for grace in the Covenant ordained our adoption. It was grace in YESHUA our SAVIOUR that has effected our redemption, our regeneration and our exaltation to heirship with YESHUA. And just as we were freely given this 'grace' we must freely give it to others.

Mr. pride serves as an admiral in satan's army and is a cruel and hurtful task master that will prevent us from speaking, thinking, or living correctly and the HEART that is absorbed in earthly affections can not be given up to GOD but rather deals in the realm of pride that deals in fear and causes panic.

Pride is satan's kind of faith and when we flatter ourselves as the devil did on the occasion that he elevated himself upward in his haughtiness, engrossed by his shrewdness to be of the opinion that he was above GOD before he fell, we too, will fall flat on our face if we lift ourselves in pride.. Do we dare set our selves up as GOD to enter excessive devotion of self worship of our own frivolous carnality? Are we not smart enough to learn from the mistakes of others who have left behind documented records for our inspection?

EPH. 2:8-10 PRIDE WILL GIVE US SPIRITUAL PRIDE AND CAUSE US TO TRUST IN OUR OWN VIRTUES RATHER THAN THE GRACE OF GOD AND THE BLOOD OF YESHUA.

MARK 12:38,39 THE SCRIBES WERE GUILTY OF PRIDE

LUKE 18:10-14 PHARISEES DEALT IN PRIDE

Intellectual pride causes one to look down with disdain on the unlearned, illiterate, oppressed, poor and down trodden. It will also cause us to look down upon our parents as out of date ignoramuses, and on our elders of our youth as back woodsy. It forgets our mental capabilities are derived from GOD.

Pride causes one to trust in material possessions, speaking only of 'myself', my this or my that, everything is mine, how great "I" am and the many places "I" have been and the many things that "I" own, forgetting that all things come from GOD. This kind of pride will cause one to parade and strut his flashy wears in front of everything and everyone so that others may admire them.

Many extravagant churches of today display social pride as it's members fancy around in their finest, glaring and envious of the wonderful dress Mrs. Smith is wearing and wondering how she can afford such luxury. Or the streamline suit Mr. Jones has on, wondering how much it cost? It is manifest in social status, class, racial rank and will caste the aire of arrogance over our countenance. It will cause us to look down upon others in our society whom we think are not socially acceptable, because of their dress, occupation or circumstances, GOD speaks to this area in

JAMES 2:1 MY BROTHERS, PRACTICE THE FAITH OF OUR LORD YESHUA {JESUS}, THE GLORIOUS MESSIAH, WITHOUT SHOWING FAVORITISM. :2 SUPPOSE A MAN COMES INTO YOUR SYNAGOGUE WEARING GOLD RINGS AND FANCY CLOTHES, AND ALSO A POOR MAN COME SIN DRESSED IN RAGS. :3 IF YOU SHOW MORE RESPECT TO THE MAN WEARING THE FANCY CLOTHES AND SAY TO HIM, "HAVE THIS GOOD SEAT HERE," WHILE TO THE POOR MAN YOU SAY, "YOU, STAND OVER THERE", OR, "SIT DOWN ON THE FLOOR BY MY FEET," :4 THEN AREN'T YOU CREATING DISTINCTIONS AMONG YOURSELVES, AND HAVEN'T YOU MADE YOURSELVES INTO JUDGES WITH EVIL MOTIVES? :5 LISTEN, MY DEAR BROTHERS, HASN'T GOD CHOSEN THE POOR OF THE WORLD TO BE RICH IN FAITH AND TO RECEIVE THE KINGDOM WHICH HE PROMISED TO THOSE WHO LOVE HIM? :6 BUT YOU DESPISE THE POOR. AREN'T THE RICH THE ONES WHO OPPRESS YOU AND DRAG YOU INTO COURT? :7 AREN'T THEY THE ONES WHO INSULT THE GOOD NAME OF HIM TO WHOM YOU BELONG? :8 IF YOU TRULY ATTAIN THE GOAL OF KINGDOM TORAH{TEACHING "LAW",

PENTATEUCH}, IN CONFORMITY WITH THE PASSAGE THAT SAYS, "LOVE YOUR NEIGHBOR AS YOURSELF," YOU ARE DOING WELL :9 BUT IF YOU SHOW FAVORITISM, YOUR ACTIONS CONSTITUTE SIN, SINCE YOU ARE CONVICTED UNDER THE TORAH AS TRANSGRESSORS. JEWISH NEW TESTAMENT

Pride of racism speeds uncontrolled through our communities today and it is a destructive evil monster that motivates assassination in the HEARTS of men and has no place in the believers life. GOD created all men equal and all have the same red blood given to them by the DIVINE CREATOR and breathe the same air. GOD has no pampered darlings and HE makes no exceptions except for those who are just in HEART.

Pride of Face is often seen as vanity and an unholy desire to display oneself. It is often the cause of immodesty.

1 TIMOTHY 2:9,10 THEY MUST POSSESS THE FORMERLY HIDDEN TRUTH OF THE FAITH WITH A CLEAN CONSCIENCE. :10 AND FIRST, LET THEM BE TESTED; THEN, IF THEY PROVE THEMSELVES BLAMELESS, LET THEM BE APPOINTED SHAMMASHIM {THOSE WHO SERVE THE CONGREGATION, DEACONS}. JEWISH NEW TESTAMENT

Pride of sin will cause one to boast of their bravery, about taking advantage of someone in an unethical or dishonest business deal. It can also cause one to lie to get away from trouble, and out of immoral pursuits. Sin causes one to be ashamed, not proud.

2 CORINTHIANS 7:10 PAIN HANDLED IN GOD'S WAY PRODUCE A TURNING FROM SIN TO GOD WHICH LEADS TO SALVATION, AND THERE IS NOTHING TO REGRET IN THAT. BUT PAIN HANDLED IN THE WORLD'S WAY PRODUCES ONLY DEATH. JEWISH NEW TESTAMENT

We must strive to possess the attitude of GOD toward pride where love is concerned.   True knowledge begets humility, not conceit and contempt. The humbling Spirit of YESHUA is the only cure for pride no matter what form it has taken. Love will cure pride and GOD is love, so without GOD we are bankrupt. We have no sufficiency in and of ourselves, our only adequacy comes from GOD alone.

PROVERBS 6:16 THESE SIX THINGS DOTH THE LORD HATE; YEA, SEVEN ARE AN ABOMINATION UNTO HIM. :17 A PROUD LOOK, A LYING TONGUE, AND HANDS THAT SHED INNOCENT BLOOD :18 AN HEART THAT DEVISETH WICKED IMAGINATIONS, FEET THAT ARE SWIFT IN RUNNING TO MISCHIEF :19 A FALSE WITNESS THAT SPEAKETH LIES, AND HE THAT SOWETH DISCORD AMONG BRETHREN.

JOHN 5:30 I CAN'T DO A THING ON MY OWN. AS I HEAR, I JUDGE; AND MY JUDGMENT IS RIGHT; BECAUSE I DON'T SEEK MY OWN DESIRE, BUT THE DESIRE OF THE ONE WHO SENT ME. JEWISH NEW TESTAMENT

We must avoid thinking of ourselves more highly than we ought to think [ROM 12:3; Gal 6:3] We must walk humbly before HIM [MIC. 6:8]   We must remember we are debtors and all that we have is given us through the grace of GOD and the help of others [1 COR. 4:7; Deut 8:11-20] We can and must come to glory only in the cross of YESHUA [GAL 6:14] We must be willing to put down our pride and crucify the flesh

NOT I, BUT CHRIST. GALATIANS 2:20

Only GOD can remove obstacles of a corrupt and tyrannizing bias that will cause our HEARTS to turn to stone and become diseased, that will eventually destroy us. Our attitude must be; Not I, but YOU, LORD bend my proud and stiff-necked "I". Help me to bow the neck and the knee and take from me the 'old man' into the 'new'. Let me behold YESHUA on Calvary, who bowed HIS Head for me and died.

48

THE RIGHT WAY
GET RIGHT OR GET LEFT

PROVERBS 14:12 THERE IS A WAY THAT SEEMS RIGHT TO A MAN BUT IN THE END IT LEADS TO DEATH.

The SCRIPTURE often speaks of life verses death, wise living verses foolish living that will push us into an early grave or a life time of walking as dead men. There will be no peace or caring for others, only deceit and greed, while grasping for another piece of this wicked world, never to be satisfied.

When we pursue the wisdom of GOD it has a tendency to transform our lives and cause us to live longer in tranquillity, peacefulness, ecstasy and the like.

When we take good times at face value too often, we don't have an opportunity to know or see behind the 'face value'. We are unable to understand that the wickedness, greed, deceit, and lies that are pushed on us in reality are evil arrows shot into our HEARTS/MINDS [intellect] by satan and/or his evil angels [demons]. In this mis understanding we seek the life styles of satan and become caught in a web which is a downward spiral into bondage. We become chained with the cords of our own sin.

PROVERBS 5:21 THE EVIL DEEDS OF A WICKED MAN ENSNARE HIM; THE CORDS OF HIS SIN HOLD HIM FAST. 22. HE WILL DIE FOR LACK OF DISCIPLINE, LED ASTRAY BY HIS OWN GREAT FOLLY.

The evil man scrambles about without eyes to see or ears to hear the ONE TRUE GOD as he dashes here and there groveling in his arrogant ignorance. His pride of life has ushered him into the throne room of the god of this depraved world and he lives with sickness and satanic miseries, under satan's suppression. Not knowing how to escape or even wishing too, because he is having a great life and is blind to the reality of his deeds. He has become as the evil one, moving under his power to do evil and think evil. He has been hoodwinked into thinking there is only one life? He is held by the cords of his sin.

By this time our systems have become completely corrupted and enemy 'ships' are floating about in our rough and stormy blood stream that is filled with the trash we have emptied into it. Our veins have given up, they are defenseless and there is nothing good left to hold too. Disease has rang the death toll and murdered any satisfactory existent delivering elements of health that were left in the system. Besides being in a major moral spiraling dilemma we have almost lost the battle for life itself. Dare we consider how GOD must grieve as HE watches our soul that HE had created for HIS service and pleasure to taken by HIS archenemy , satan. We are on pride alert, heading for a fall.

The BIBLE'S conception of life and death mean more than survival of our bodies. To live for GOD means to live in abundance which is "genuine living" occupied with soundness of mind and body, contentment, happiness and intelligence. The LORD'S honour, ability, holiness, graciousness and faithfulness to the believer is demonstrated through faith. There is an unreserved confidence because of GOD'S nature that HE will lead, guide and deliver us from the enemy.

Faith toward GOD is the committal of life to HIM [LUKE 23:46]. The act and confession of faith strengthens trust and accentuates the difference between truth and falsity. [JOHN 2:8]. Faith, believes and lays hold upon things not yet seen.

Sin equates sickness and is the agency for spiritual and physical decay. As a dead man the body walks about with cancer or some other life menacing disease eating at the bones, hardening the arteries and HEART. Perpetual impending doom subscribed by satan fabricating assignments for our expiration that only THE SUPREME BEING has the authority to void. The person who is spiritually deceased has bypassed the path of prudence, because GOD is wisdom and they are as good as extinguished even though they promenade around.

1 TIMOTHY 5:6 BUT SHE [OR HE] THAT LIVETH IN PLEASURE IS DEAD ALREADY.

Anytime we step out of GOD'S WILL, HIS Natural Order is upset. Since we are made in HIS Image only HIS ORDER is good. Our movement away from HIS WILL automatically brings about dilemmas in our system that is produced and organized by the DIVINE CREATOR. When we move away from HIS Will for our life we step into satan's dominion and divine manifestation, instantly our position becomes dangerously uncertain. We become temperamental and unstable in our ways and our bodies that are created in HIS Image become challenged by satan's un-natural lethargy. The devil is a as a roaring lion seeking to devour us. JOHN 10:10 "satan COMES TO STEAL, KILL AND DESTROY" all that GOD has made and given to us in HIS Glorious Image.

JOHN 10:10 THE THIEF [satan] COMETH NOT BUT TO STEAL, KILL, AND TO DESTROY; I AM COME THAT THEY MIGHT HAVE LIFE, AND THAT THEY MIGHT HAVE IT MORE ABUNDANTLY.

GOD IS PERFECT IN ALL HIS WAYS AND ATTRIBUTES, IN HIM IS NO GUILE. Our bodies develop guile through serving satan. Though we are created by GOD, we commence to promote depression, disease and apprehension that eventually runs into plague and death, we have allowed the devil to seize authority of our system.

PSALMS 31:12 I AM FORGOTTEN AS A DEAD MAN OUT OF MIND; I AM LIKE A BROKEN VESSEL.

The cultural baggage of life's pressures have become heavy and bankrupt traditions weigh us down when we seek self indulgence. Instead of seeking renewal through HIS WORD for our minds, we turn to superficial sparks that are only temporary such as a bandied. We exist in cultural adultery that denies the healing saving powers of GOD and therefore deny any super natural works of GOD.

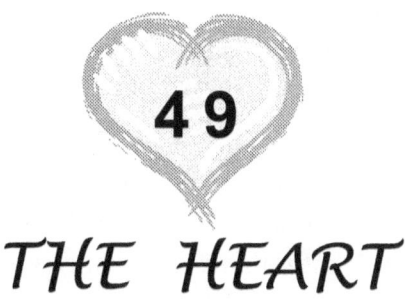

THE HEART

The HEART is the chief organ of any physical body and in mankind it is the place GOD searches. Thus the conscience {moral responsibility} holds the abiding truth in human life. The HEART is the hidden spring of our peculiar existence. It occupies the most important place in the mortal system and is responsible for man's complete mental and moral activity. It holds emotions, reasons and will, rational and/or emotional.

1 PETER 3:4 BUT LET IT BE THE HIDDEN MAN OF THE HEART IN THAT WHICH IS NOT CORRUPTIBLE, EVEN THE ORNAMENT OF A MEEK AND QUIET SPIRIT, WHICH IS IN THE SIGHT OF GOD OF GREAT PRICE.

We are made in the "image and likeness" of GOD. This likeness to GOD lies in the fact that man is meant to be a personal, rational, and moral being. Even so men possess only a small amount of the traits of GOD'S personality. GOD fashioned man in HIS own likeness but we have no capability to understand, love or forgive as GOD has and only through HIM can we bear witness or acquire a degree of these characteristics.

ECCL. 3:11b GOD HATH SET THE WORLD IN MAN'S HEART, SO THAT NO MAN CAN FIND OUT THE WORK THAT GOD MAKETH FROM THE BEGINNING TO THE END.

The world appeals to the HEART of a Christian through the lust of the flesh, the lust of the eyes, and the pride of life.. When first we are effected we will lose our enjoyment of the FATHER'S love and our desire to do HIS WILL. The BIBLE will become boring and prayer a difficult chore. Even Christian fellowship will seem empty and disappointing. It is not that something is wrong with others and certainly not the GOSPEL, it is our HEART, it has began to reject Righteousness. If we are well-acquainted with GOD'S WORD when the world seizes us in one of these regions we will promptly recognize his trickery and if we are discerning we will hasten our restoration to SCRIPTURE in compelling rapidity to gain back ground the enemy has stolen.

But how many are not familiar with lucifer's insidious chicanery and take part in his evil domain ignorant of his intentions to STEAL, KILL AND DESTROY. Perhaps they have not even understood or heard about the extraordinary love of YESHUA and how HE signifies victory for the prisoner? How many disregard GOD'S way only to sink into the cesspool of hell because we failed to demonstrate SALVATION to them?

GOD is all knowing, there is not anything that transpires that HE does not fully comprehend and is not sovereign over, and that encompass the enemies afflictions, battles, treachery, and the like. "We" can not fathom or comprehend the intensity of THE FATHERS love that HE felt for us as HE sent HIS SON as sacrifice for our sin. How many of us could treasure another so much that we would be willing to give one of our children or an only child to die for them? Yet HIS affection for us was so great that HE sent HIS Only SON. And what about the SON? How could HE have such devotion for us that HE would submit to death on our behalf? Why? Should we not ask ourselves? Yet we will all encounter and one day join HIM in HIS Glory if we hold fast to HIS WORD and embellish HIS WILL in obedience and faith.

REV. 7:16-17 THEY SHALL HUNGER NO MORE, NEITHER THIRST ANY MORE; NEITHER SHALL THE SUN LIGHT ON THEM, NOR ANY HEAT. 17. FOR THE LAMB WHICH IS IN THE MIDST OF THE THRONE SHALL FEED THEM, AND SHALL LEAD THEM UNTO LIVING FOUNTAINS OF WATER AND GOD SHALL WIPE AWAY ALL TEARS FORM THEIR EYES.

Peace is found where it is lost, in human attitudes and behavior. It is easy to find peace in the good natured disposition that pursues the principals of the LORD. The enjoyment of good days is not an accident; it is an achievement. The pleasant life is always conditional and one of the conditions is the pursuit of peace.   Peace and pleasantness just go together in a cause and effect relationship in which each promotes the other; and the result is the enhancement of health. So if we want health and happiness, we must seek peace and pursue it. Forbearance is an additive to peace with in one's HEART and to achieve that tranquil life, we must be charitable. We must learn to be kind and forgive others as we have been forgiven.

1 PETER 3:10,11 FOR HE THAT WILL LOVE LIFE AND SEE GOOD DAYS. LET HIM SEEK PEACE AND ENSURE IT.

PSALMS 145:9   THE LORD IS GOOD TO ALL; AND HIS TENDER MERCIES ARE OVER ALL HIS WORKS.

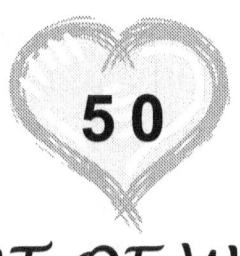

50

HEART OF WORLD

America's sin is inscribed upon HER HEART and the penal fires so hot, will be ever lasting. She has become the harlot in total disregard for GOD'S Law while clinging tightly to the genius of man and human forms of security. The intellect of man has replaced our confidence in GOD. Aggrandized by the archenemy of our spiritual being human intelligence grandstands as a masterpiece to satan at the height of hypocrisy and egotistism. Love of money, success or reputation are all dazzling illusions of mastery and triumph that mankind has stubbornly set up as counterfeit idols of adoration.

ROMANS 3:13-18 THEIR THROATS ARE OPEN GRAVES, THEY USE THEIR TONGUES TO DECEIVE. VIPERS' VENOM IS UNDER THEIR LIPS. :14 THEIR MOUTHS ARE FULL OF CURSES AND BITTERNESS. :15 THEIR FEET RUSH TO SHED BLOOD. :16 IN THEIR WAYS ARE RUIN AND MISERY :17 AND THE WAY OF SHALOM {PEACE} THEY DO NOT KNOW. :18 THERE IS NO FEAR OF GOD BEFORE THEIR EYES.

America's death is eminent without GOD, this great nation will fall from within and wonder why? Her blindness is overwhelming. But GOD'S people have the promise of forever from an eternal living GOD. Do we dare run the risk of liberty which stakes all upon GOD alone? Do we dare walk by faith as we are instructed?

The spirit of compromise and conformity reigns today, the humble simplicity of YESHUA has been laid aside for pomp, prideful traditions of man that substitute human theories for the requirements of GOD.

The god of this world has gained possession of man's HEART and formed traditions, opinion and prejudices against the beauty of GOD'S WORKS. Mankind is one of GOD'S most cherished works and those who find fault in others are actually condemning themselves. One's fault finding is an index to their own personal problems thus in one's habitual condemnations of others the true character of their self is revealed.

2 CORINTHIANS 4:4 IN WHOM THE god OF THIS WORLD HATH BLINDED THE MINDS OF THEM, WHICH BELIEVE NOT, LEST THE LIGHT OF THE GLORIOUS GOSPEL OF CHRIST, WHO IS THE IMAGE OF GOD, SHOULD SHINE UNTO THEM.

We have become so pre-occupied with the meditation and distress of self, coupled with the urgency of this world until contention has filled our memory and we have neither the time nor spirit to see GOD'S Hand at work. The enemy has prevailed by launching noxious clouds to shroud our mental balance with insignificant thoughts and events.

Utterances denoting GOD'S wrath encompass this world more frequently in form of storms, famines, murders and the like, while the majority of our leaders are insidious and emphatic as they study to compose duplicity and concealment in their defense, for their own vain glories.

We live in an age of vengeance, anger, passion and wrath and most of our contemporaries have no awareness of the meaning of these signs that GOD'S wrath is pouring out upon us because they are unable to conceive GOD'S warnings. America has provoked GOD'S anger by Her impassivity and indifference where the Blood of infants scream up from the ground for justice and the responsibility belongs to every confirmed believer to deliver a reflection of YESHUA in everyday life, and stand to hold high GOD'S STANDARD.

1 CORINTHIANS 1:29 THAT NO FLESH SHOULD GLORY IN HIS PRESENCE.

There is nothing certain or good about any thing lest the HOLY SPIRIT is working from the HEART and our actions and motives are seated in GOD'S Will and for HIS purpose. We must apply and make good use of everything for the benefit of others as a reflection of YESHUA, for nothing we do here in this life will benefit another or even be remembered unless it to further the KINGDOM OF OUR LORD.

We were not born for ourselves but for GOD'S pleasure and our business is to do good and to think good and pure thoughts in HIS WILL. We are to protect our intellect which bears passage to our HEART to make sure that no bizarre hostile alien enters to obstruct our system or incite unsoundness. In consummating a tranquil moral sense we will have a GOD-given tranquilizer better than medicine.

1 CORINTHIANS 13:6 REJOICE NOT IN INIQUITY, BUT REJOICETH IN THE TRUTH.

In this life we are in a state of trial and probation as OUR SOUL & HEART is being adapted for Eternity, every life will count no matter how big or how small. We will be rewarded for the choices we have made in this lifetime in other words the opportunity of accomplishing what ever we choose will determine infinity. We must cling to YESHUA and HIS WORD for encouragement, for health and for faith. Fear, anxiety, grief, and gloom are results of doubt, disbelief and distrust. These HEART disturbances can only be dispelled by faith in YESHUA.

As the DIVINE CREATOR assembled us HE issued to each a free will and expected us to act according to HIS Image because HE implanted knowledge of right and wrong within the frame work of all. By HIS design everyone will experience an equal share of misery and will be responsible for how these miseries are allowed to affect us. As miseries begin to spring up as weeds into a flower garden on all sides we learn to deal with them by means of what GOD has given us. Be it other persons or our own problems we must learn that patience is an asset meant to be given out to others as well as ourselves. Forgiveness is a tranquilizer that will settle nerves and a stimulant which invigorates health.

Peace with self and with others comes in the graceful handling of little annoyances and elimination of the little weeds of impatience that spring up from time to time. For even though the weeds of impatience are small and even un-noticeable, when left unattended they will grow into large and ugly noxious invasive plants that add new miniature crops daily. As they appear and are left uninterrupted before long they seize authority and begin to control and embitter the character, destroy peace, create anxiety and make our associations with others almost intolerable, which should otherwise be sweet and peaceable.

1 PETER 1:16 BECAUSE IT IS WRITTEN, BE YE HOLY;   FOR I AM HOLY

Each Individual Being involves a Trinity made up of body, soul and spirit that are finite, having limits to their strengths, thoughts, abilities, etc. It is in knowing GOD and seeking HIS wisdom that we overcome satan's dominion. A faithful follower who loves

GOD with all their HEART and is set to know YESHUA and HIS FATHER'S WILL without a doubt, will be inundated by demons sent from the prince of darkness for the purpose of capturing the soul for his evil aspirations. These demonic employees will be accessible in all forms, but most particularly in the regions we are most exposed. If we carry through in GOD'S WORD we will be shielded by GODLY Angels and after a period this monarch of hell will tire and pull his army away for another strategy of attack. Most likely the other tactic will include overwhelming and inflaming our children or those we most love and cherish.. We must learn to speak each morning, in the early hours to our HEAVENLY FATHER and plea the Precious BLOOD OF YESHUA over them for their defense, whether we are in their favor or not. We must be sure to petition GOD to render null and void all of satan's assignments for ourselves as well as those we care for.

1 CORINTHIANS 1:25 BECAUSE THE FOOLISHNESS OF GOD IS WISER THAN MEN; AND THE WEAKNESS OF GOD IS STRONGER THAN MEN.

GOD'S Trinity is made up of FATHER, SON AND HOLY SPIRIT [GHOST] which is infinite; meaning HE is very great, lacking limits, endless, immeasurable and vast. HE was before time and shall be for all eternity. HIS existence is the greatest and most profound idea the human mind can ever conceivably entertain. We can each experience a personal GOD, WHO cares for us, watches over us, grieves over our demented decisions but loves us none the less, WHOSE love is unconditional and astounding.

All mankind has some idea of a supreme Being. This argument has often been challenged but never refuted. While the concepts of GOD found among many cultures and civilizations differ greatly on the number, name, and nature of the supreme Being, nevertheless the idea remains. A classic example of this is the amazing story of Helen Keller {1880-1968}. From the age of two, Miss Keller was blind, deaf and without the sense of smell. After months of agonizing and fruitless attempts on the part of her teacher to communicate with this young girl, a miracle occurred. One day Helen suddenly understood the concept and meaning of running water! From this humble foundation Miss Keller built a lofty tower of thought, including the ability to use her voice in speaking. She became an educated and articulate human being. Sometime after she had progressed to the point that she could engage in conversation, she was told of GOD and HIS love in sending YESHUA to die on the cross. She is said to have responded with joy, "I always knew HE was there, but I didn't know HIS NAME!"

ROMANS 8:27 HE THAT SEARCHETH THE HEARTS KNOWETH WHAT IS THE MIND OF THE SPIRIT, BECAUSE HE MAKETH INTERCESSION FOR THE SAINTS ACCORDING TO THE WILL OF GOD.

Wellness is synonymous with Obedience and Obedience is a stewardship of faith from the HEART. Faith is moving forward in righteousness, believing what GOD has said will happen. We are unable in our human {limited} form to see or realize the possible end, for to us it seems impossible. There are no short cuts, life is like a race. The difference is in the position we hold as we run. Paul often compared life to athletics. Good athletes demonstrate how we must approach the everyday gridiron. With devotion - committed love for the tasks themselves. With direction - an eye for where we're headed. With determination - endurance built upon intestinal fortitude and with discipline - a patient plodding that doesn't let the tail wag the dog.

Rabbits that run way ahead and take long breaks never out do the slow going but persistent turtles. We must be a turtle with rabbit legs and coach ourselves to stay in GOD'S WILL. Not to run far ahead of HIM or slack off and fall behind, always quick to reflect HIS character and disposition of righteousness and forgiveness. No matter if another should clip us, punch us, stomp our toes, call us names, scare us, question or laugh at us we must continuously tread in the consciousness of mercy. As we pursue and embrace GOD'S exoneration for ourselves, we must constantly be prepared to pardon others, for we allow unforgiveness to accumulate it will hoard filthy rags in the HEART that will soon become a mountain of retaliation that will suffocate or strangle the righteous clean clothes to overtake the HEART with jealousy and bitterness. The acquisition of these traits leads to withdrawal, selfishness and dis-ease that will establish walls of death.

MATTHEW 19:26 BUT YESHUA {JESUS} BEHELD THEM AND SAID UNTO THEM, WITH MEN THIS IS IMPOSSIBLE, BUT WITH GOD ALL THINGS ARE POSSIBLE.

Our entire system is blessed or defiled by what our HEART is filled with and the choice of blessings or defilement is of our own choosing. A defiled HEART will cause corrosion, decay and hardening. By giving priority to spiritual things we are overwhelmed by a tremendous driving power to eliminate negative thoughts that burn energy and waste time such as doubt, faultfinding, hate, selfishness, vengeance and unforgiveness. The obedient believer replenishes negative qualities with emphatic but unique traits that strengthen faith, love, tolerance, unselfishness, magnanimity and forgiveness. They are cautious to influence energies from the wasteland of fatalistic reasoning to the confident channels of organization and accomplishment. Consequently shedding light on why honorableness is a good investment. Righteousness is affiliated to the providential care of GOD and establishes an enterprise strategy so efficient and immense that it includes the responsibility of both man and GOD and extents all the way from earth to heaven.

PROVERBS 13:12 HOPE DEFERRED MAKETH THE HEART SICK.

PROVERBS 13:13 WHOSOEVER DESPISETH THE WORD SHALL BE DESTROYED.

The enemy satan will be on earth until GOD'S timing has passed for him to go into the pit that GOD prepared for him and his followers. But no one can afford to relax as satan compounds and bombard his corrupt arrows of thoughtlessness into our sanity and HEART. This armed conflict will continue as long as we are flesh and blood, but what we consume and adopt to embrace from this monarch of hell will determine if we will see Salvation or damnation for it was YESHUA who instructed us to "BE HOLY AS HE IS HOLY".

Our testimony will be seen and understood according to the sincerity of our HEART. It should favor a likeness of YESHUA and be cherished, prepared, well-proportioned and attentive to risks to be considered as authentic. PROV. 25:26 tells us that a Righteous man who gives way to wickedness is like a muddied spring or a polluted well. This Jekyll/Hyde performance is not so unusual in the present as many phony baloneys dramatize in every theater of life. We can be confident that hypocrisy earns a loudly amusing disrespect from the world as well as from the MESSIAH. When we gait about as a hypocrite and communicate as a charlatan it is confirmation to the world that righteousness is no different than the social milieu and motivated thoughts that there is no incentive to fancy GOD'S RIGHTEOUSNESS.

MATTHEW 15:19 FOR OUT OF THE HEART PROCEED EVIL THOUGHTS, MURDERS, ADULTERIES, FORNICATION'S, THEFTS, FALSE WITNESS, BLASPHEMIES. 20. THESE ARE THE THINGS WHICH DEFILE A MAN;

Scripture regards our HEART as a sphere of influence {power to effect others} but we are not to stand in judgment. We have not been given that right except by GOD'S Spirit, to call to task another who professes GOD in his speech but denies The LORD in his affairs.. Even then we are to be examples, speaking only in love and only when prompted by GOD'S HOLY SPIRIT. For it is only by the SPIRIT of the LORD that we can be effective, for in our flesh and prideful speaking we offer nothing.

When we are swift to speak in our flesh we usurp the HOLY SPIRIT'S path, HEARTS become hardened and GOD'S SPIRIT is rejected. The key is to let the BIBLE master us and not spend our energies in mastering the BIBLE for it will put both a fire and a song in our HEART when we read it and heed its tremendous truths. But to master the doctrine of GOD'S WORD is impossible and as useless as arguing about how many angels can dance on the head of a pen? Or thinking GOD would create a rock so heavy that HE could not move it? One who indulges in such arguments are as far removed from GOD'S WILL and truth as the Babe in the manger at Bethlehem is from Rudolph the Red-nosed reindeer.

ROMANS 2:15 WHO SHOW THE WORK OF THE LAW WRITTEN IN THEIR HEARTS, THEIR CONSCIENCE ALSO BEARING WITNESS, AND THEIR THOUGHTS THE MEANWHILE ACCUSING OR ELSE EXCUSING ONE ANOTHER.

Each of us have a moral conscience and knowledge to determine the difference between 'the act of good' or the 'act of evil' and it's value, truth and reality. Conscience will infallibly accuse or acquit us. On the day we stand before our Creator, all our secrets will be read and judged by YESHUA. We will not be seated beside HIM to judge but will be judged, excused or damned for what we have allowed to be written on our HEART.

On that day divine righteous judgment will be manifest and each of us will see our lives mirrored according to our works and at that moment our eternal destinies will be forever set. If our works have been by faith, entwined with patience, well doing, seeking GOD and HIS WILL, then results will be eternal life. But works of disobedience and wickedness will culminate in a firey pit of wrath and fury where trouble and anguish will be spread over every soul who has worked evil. Impartiality of the divine judgment will be demonstrated and none will be exempt.

Cleansing of the HEART comes by trusting in GOD through YESHUA, and is the one and only condition for SALVATION. When redemption is unearthed in the HEART we are quickly humbled and eager to bend the knee in regret and repentance for our past transgression. Haughtiness is put away with sin and a gentle and kind loving spirit finds residence, one who communicates with compassionate words and behavior that will not be found condemning the down trodden but stepping beside them as examples in commitment and procedure as a reflection of YESHUA.

PROVERBS 23:9 SPEAK NOT IN THE EARS OF A FOOL: FOR HE WILL DESPISE THE WISDOM OF THY WORDS. 10. REMOVE NOT THE OLD LANDMARK; AND ENTER NOT INTO THE FIELDS OF THE FATHERLESS; 11. FOR THEIR REDEEMER IS MIGHTY; HE SHALL PLEAD THEIR CAUSE WITH THEE.

Our LORD'S rule is the same purport "GIVE NOT THAT WHICH IS HOLY UNTO THE DOGS; NEITHER CAST YE YOUR PEARLS BEFORE SWINE, LEST THEY TRAMPLE THEM UNDER FOOT, AND TURN AGAIN AND REND YOU" MATTHEW 7:6

In essence GOD has instructed us not to cast our good instruction upon the incorrigible sinners unless there be any hope of reclaiming the fool, thus we should make every effort for his precious soul , to tell him about the love of YESHUA. Speaking in the SPIRIT of our MASTER, prepared through HIS WORD and enthusiastic about introducing the GOSPEL to the worst and the most unwilling, and being cautious to never make the rule of common sense the excuse for habitual idleness. Yet there is a time to keep silent as well as a time to speak and such a time we shall understand by the trial to our own spirit. Often we long to speak in compassion but self denial, not self indulgence, restrains. We have been told 'SPEAK NOT IN THE EARS OF A FOOL' for instead of being thankful for the instruction, he will despise the wisdom of our words. The safe rule is never to speak without prayer for divine guidance and simplicity and love.

To many of us take for granted the rank of GOD'S HOLY SPIRIT and move forward in our flesh when we really should be prayerfully petitioning GOD to dispatch ministering angels to witness GOD'S LOVE through us to others. We must endeavor to discern GOD'S discretion for our walk, our conversation, and our procedure. Often the HOLY SPIRIT foreordains us as a witness to others through our walk rather then testimony and as they observe our inner peace and joy, their longing will be re-channeled in the direction of YESHUA as the HOLY SPIRIT prepares the HEART.

If we speak in pride, desiring to show how learned we are, we accomplish nothing thus our fine eloquent words are empty. For it is by our illustration, through our conduct and from a compassionate HEART that is skilled to communicate to the destitute and tormented HEART of others, that will touch and be effective to guide another to the LORD. But even than the flesh must be fed and clothed before the ear can listen because most who are destitute and lost do not care what we know, only what we can do for them.

They are able only to see what is before them and thus our words mean nothing unless they are from the HEART. When our HEART is prepared to do GOD'S Will we will love them in deed first, realizing the enemy satan has entered and supplemented his evil traits of rejection, to stir up their pain of being unloved and unwanted.

Articulating knowledge from GOD'S WORD is a talent to be wisely published but not promiscuously. There should be no concealment of fundamental truth in declaring a suitable occasion, or in speaking to suitable persons the gracious dealings of GOD. However much harm can be done by intruding on the ungodly those interior matters of our experiences from our HEART because their HEART is unprepared to hear. Every truth is not always fit for every person or for every time.

ECCLESIATES 3:7 A TIME TO REND, AND A TIME TO SEW; A TIME TO KEEP SILENCE AND A TIME TO SPEAK.

YESHUA charged HIS Disciples with the prudent concealment of knowledge after HIS example, till a more favorable season, the right time. What is time? Aging does not wait on it, songwriters write lyric about it, writers make poems about it. Philosophers theorize it, everybody waste it, clocks click right past it, prisoners spend it, dancers promenade to it, New Year promises it, travelers try to make it, daylight savings time tries to save it, the elderly speculate about where it went, kids wonder why it moves so slowly and graduates ponder on what it holds. Time advances as opportunities come and go, yet the only genuine time that shapes a difference is the time we give to THE LORD..

Time is priceless and as it advances we will never again be able to repossess it or retreat to it. Such are our words after they have departed from our mouth we can at no time take them back to resay them in a kinder way perhaps. GOD has made each of us the administrator of our time and we must disburse it wisely and be sure not to squander it as the slothful one who is enamored with his bed of ease. He influences himself as the hinges upon the door. Moving indeed but making no progress, he works from one excuse to the next. From year to year he is moving as he swings forward and then backward. Always beginning but never finishing; determining nothing, with no HEART for exertion only complaining.

MATTHEW. 16:20 THEN CHARGED HE HIS DISCIPLES THAT THEY SHOULD TELL NO MAN THAT HE WAS YESHUA THE MESSIAH.

EXAMPLES:

[1] The Apostle concealed his knowledge for fourteen years, and even then mentioned it reluctantly, to vindicate his own rightful claims of Apostleship. 2 COR. 12:1-6

[2] Elihu, though "full of matter", and longing to give vent, yet prudently concealed his knowledge, till his elders had opened his way.
JOB 33:6,18,19.

[3] Abraham spared the feelings of his family, and cleared his own path, by hiding the dreadful message of his GOD. GEN. 22:1-7

[4] Joseph concealed his kindred for the discipline of his brethren GEN. 42:7

[5] Esther concealed her origin as a Hebrew from a prudent regard of consequences to herself ESTH 2:10

[6] JEREMIAH answered all that he was bound to speak; not all that he might have spoken. JERE. 38:24-27

While there is nothing that will justify speaking contrary to truth, we are not always obliged to tell the whole truth, "the wise man's HEART will discern both time and judgment" and it will cherish sound judgment and ardent love for truth, with out zealousness to move ahead out of GOD'S WILL. The wise will seek GOD in every area.

Patience is the a peace-maker. Soft and healing words gain a double victory over ourselves and to whom we speak. As we speak healing-encouraging words we are blessed by the GOD of health. Wisdom is proved not by quantum of knowledge, but by its right application. The right use of knowledge distinguishes the wise.

2 TIMOTHY 2:15 WORKMAN APPROVED OF GOD THAT NEEDETH NOT TO BE ASHAMED

Too often the want of knowledge gives out truth loosely and unsuitably, as to open, rather than to shut, the mouth of the gainsayer. This brings discredit upon the truth rather than conviction to the adversary. The tongue of the wise directs right application of knowledge when the HOLY SPIRIT is in control. May we not ever find ourselves guilty of forgetting our own feeble infancy so that we can not reach down to remove the thorn out of our brother tender feet.

HEBREWS 12;13 LEST THAT WHICH IS LAMED BE TURNED OUT OF THE WAY; BUT RATHER LET IT BE HEALED.

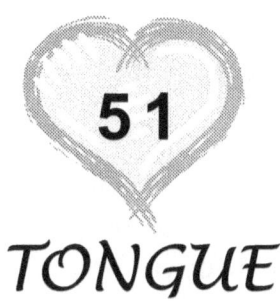

TONGUE

JAMES 3:4 THINK OF A SHIP, ALTHOUGH IT IS HUGE AND IS DRIVEN BY STRONG WINDS, YET THE PILOT CAN STEER IT WHEREVER HE WANTS WITH JUST A SMALL RUDDER. :5 SO TOO THE TONGUE IS A TINY PART OF THE BODY, YET IT BOASTS GREAT THINGS. SEE HOW A LITTLE FIRE SETS A WHOLE FOREST ABLAZE. :6 YES, THE TONGUE IS A FIRE, A WORLD OF WICKEDNESS. THE TONGUE IS SO PLACED IN OUR BODY THAT IT DEFILES EVERY PART OF IT, SETTING ABLAZE THE WHOLE OF OUR LIFE; AND IT IS SET ON FIRE BY GEY-HINNOM {HELL} ITSELF. JEWISH NEW TESTAMENT

May we walk in abundant life and be wise enough to heed the power house with in so that our tongue may be disciplined and consecrated. There are some among us who say they can hold their tongues and others who admit they can not but unless we are faithful Believers of GOD'S WORD we are controlled by the devil and therefore incapable of speaking in wisdom. Words are one of the most powerful additives in this world. YESHUA was the WORD INCARNATE. Life is in the WORD. GOD releases HIS Faith in WORDS. YESHUA spoke GOD'S WORD continually and HE established GOD'S WORD. Our words work to issue bondage against us or blessings for us. GOD has told us in HIS WORD that our words are kept in HIS BOOK of REMEMBRANCE to be used for or against us when judgment comes.

ECCL. 8:5 BECAUSE TO EVERY PURPOSE THERE IS TIME AND JUDGMENT, THEREFORE THE MISERY OF MAN IS GREAT UPON HIM.

Often circumstances may prudently dictate concealment of our words, our thoughts but in our zeal for GOD we blurt out GOD'S WORD in our own wisdom, and may cause more hurt than good. Our good intentions are side tracked. For many of us, to frequently we program our vocabulary with the devil's rhetoric, attempting to 'fit in' or 'be cool'. We have pronounced affliction, misery and death into the vocabulary and they have taken root in the HEART which sends them to the intellect where they become a demonstration of reality and exhibit the true character.

ACTS 15:8 GOD, WHICH KNOWETH THE HEARTS, BARE WITNESS, GIVING THEM THE HOLY SPIRIT EVEN AS HE DID US.

To the true believer holiness is not merely a matter of external observances or precise keeping of rules but a HEART attitude toward GOD that tends to keep our HEART healthy. It is not in the letter of the law that GOD looks at and is concerned with but the spirit that we keep hidden within our HEART. We need to be aware of what GOD'S WORD says about the mouth and the tongue;

PROVERBS 10:11 ""THE MOUTH OF A RIGHTEOUS MAN IS A WELL OF LIFE"

PROVERBS 10:21 THE LIPS OF THE RIGHTEOUS FEED MANY; BUT FOOLS DIE FOR WANT OF WISDOM. THE FEAR OF THE WICKED, IT SHALL COME UPON HIM; BUT THE DESIRES OF THE RIGHTEOUS SHALL BE GRANTED.

Wit, originality, imagination may supply the feast of reason, and the overflowing of soul but how short lived and poor is this pleasure compared with the godly instruction. The fool despises discretion and falls victim to his own folly, his mouth is covered with confusion consequently his fear activates an attack from the prince of darkness. Wise men lay up knowledge for their own use but fools lay it out. For want of sound wisdom, they open their mouths for their own mischief in profane rebellion, groveling selfishness, ungodly worldliness or hateful pride. But because GOD is patient, HE is long-suffering and endures the mockery of mankind as they stand out like monuments against HIS Holiness and HIS WILL. The evil of a HEART always exposes itself with external observances that are a perversion and strictly condemned by YESHUA {JESUS} in:

MATTHEW 15:6b THUS HAVE YE MADE THE COMMANDMENT OF GOD OF NO EFFECT BY YOUR TRADITIONS.

The self centered individual is the unhappiest person in the world with a spectacular consciousness of self that is continually focused on their own inward, egocentric appetite and self satisfaction. Their agenda is built totally around 'self' and their greed can not be satisfied. They are sightless to the hunger or even the neediness or others on every side of them. How desolate and contemptible they will be when they grow older as they casually push others away to promote their own programs. Getting out of self will take the emptiness out of one's life and fill it with delight that magnifies health. Just as the little flower seed never becomes beautiful and fragrant until it breaks out of itself and grows up and blossoms, so it is with man. Until he breaks out of himself he can not flourish, grow or know GOD.

In 1 Peter 3:4 The HEART is described as the hidden man that lies unseen and deep within and needs to have access to the "SON" for a healthy balance. GOD prefers to see beauty of character which will never fade and can not be worn as a cloak or a piece of jewelry or the wearing of hair in a certain way, etc.

1 PETER 3:4 BUT LET IT BE THE HIDDEN MAN OF THE HEART IN THAT WHICH IS NOT CORRUPTIBLE, EVEN THE ORNAMENT OF A MEEK AND QUIET SPIRIT, WHICH IS IN THE SIGHT OF GOD OF GREAT PRICE.

A gentle and quiet spirit is one which gently puts up with the impositions of others without causing any itself. Such a character is a witness to a pure and good conscience as it testifies to good pedigree within the people of GOD and brings joyful satisfactions into man's turbulent HEART. There is no rest like the peace in the house of one's own conscience.

THERE IS NO PILLOW SO SOFT AS A CLEAR

CONSCIENCE.

FRENCH PROVERB

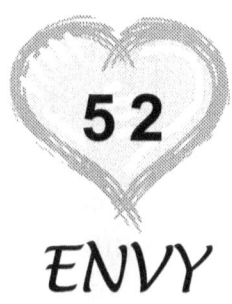

ENVY

Envy is the deadly fruit of selfishness. It will be wounded by the neighbors prosperity and will find pleasure in his associates ruin or injury.   It is an implacable passion with a fearful train of evils.. Reasonable answers or opinions only operate as the oil to fan the flame rather than the water to quench it. Just as grievous words are the oil that stirs up the fire, the soft tongue and kind words are the water to quench. Even so man's natural propensity is to feed the angry flame rather than quench it because the spirit of flesh is the characteristic spirit of this world and it is a habitual enemy to the HOLY SPIRIT. The natural man has no authority or power over the spirit of flesh, thus strife and envy is born and the HEART is always effected. Harbored envy will cause strife to the HEART to damn the soul and it is a common sin yet seldom confessed. Anger is stirred by offense; envy is stirred by godliness, prosperity or favor.

Socrates said "Envy is the daughter of pride, the author of murder and revenge, the begetter of secret sedition, the perpetual tormentor of virtue. Envy is the filthy slime of the soul; a venom, a poison, a quicksilver, which consumeth the flesh and drieth up the marrow of the bones".

Defined: Webster says "Envy is discontent at the excellence or good fortune of another; resentful, begrudging" These conditions are alien to our Spirit and body and will cause discomfort, stress and eventually disease.

JAMES 3:14,15 SAYS ENVY IS EARTHY, SENSUAL AND DEVILISH.

PSALMS 37:1; 73:3; PROVERBS 24:1,19; 23:17 SAYS ENVY IS INSIDIOUS.

Cruden Concordance says "Discontent at the excellence or good fortune of another. The BIBLE explains it as the distinct idea of malice or spite. The revisions often replace it by jealousy". To envy is to eye the subject with evil intent.

Lord Clarendon says, "Envy is a weed that grows in all soils and climates".

Envy renders its victims miserable and unhappy. It is a disease of the soul hidden in the HEART that if left alone to feed and cultivate will eventually destroy.

PROVERBS 14:30 A SOUND HEART IS THE LIFE OF THE FLESH; ENVY IS ROTTENNESS TO THE BONES.

Envy is a cancer that eats away at the bone as malignancy. It is leprosy to the flesh and death to our spiritual life. The envious HEARTED will be tempted to defame the character and jeopardize the influence of the envied. GOD strictly prohibits us against envy, advising us to put away envy as we would discard filthy clothing. [1 PETER 2:1; GAL 5:26; ROM. 13:13]

Who can stand before envy? When lucifer lost his place as one of the three Archangels it was for envy of GOD, his CREATOR. And he [satan] was hurled out of Heaven, he envied man and ceased not to work his destruction thus the perfect innocence of paradise fell before envy. Envy shed the first human blood that ever stained the ground between Cain and Abel. We must remember that sin shall not have dominion but the struggle is sharp to the end.

The natural man will look at grace with an envious eye because they do not know the LORD. They will strive to darken the lives that outshine their own and defame holiness for they have no HEART to follow. But those who have true worth that only comes from a relationship with GOD in themselves can never envy others.

GOD will reward us according to what we cherish in our HEART.

2 TIMOTHY 2:24 AND THE SERVANT OF THE LORD MUST NOT STRIVE, BUT BE GENTLE UNTO ALL MEN, APT TO TEACH, PATIENT. 25. IN MEEKNESS, INSTRUCTING THOSE THAT OPPOSE HIM, IF GOD PERHAPS, WILL GIVE THEM REPENTANCE TO THE ACKNOWLEDGE OF THE TRUTH.

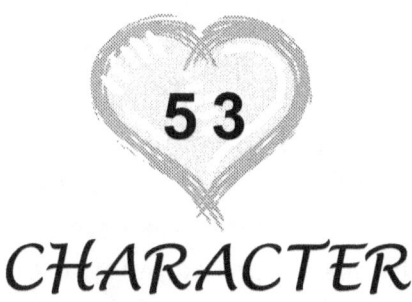

CHARACTER

The HEART represents the true character of each of us but conceals it.   When we are obedient to HIS natural laws we will desire to know HIM and will grow to understand HIS treasures through HIS Written WORD. HIS moral law will be our guide and we will reflect the attributes of HIS character. Even the heathen will recognize the peace, wisdom and strength that comes from our HEART as that of the wisdom of a living GOD. One of the most necessary conditions of contented living and sound health is an untroubled conscience which is a fountainhead for happiness through the feeling of peace. Peace with one's self, peace with one's record and peace with GOD.

JAMES 3:17 BUT THE WISDOM THAT IS FROM ABOVE IS FIRST PURE, THEN PEACEABLE, GENTLE, AND EASY TO BE ENTREATED,   FULL OF MERCY AND GOOD FRUITS, WITHOUT PARTIALITY, AND WITHOUT HYPOCRISY.

No man can impart that which he himself has not received. In the work of GOD, humanity can originate nothing. No man can by his own effort make himself a light bearer for GOD. It is the golden oil emptied by the heavenly messengers that produces a continuous, bright and shining light. Only love from GOD continually transferred to man, will enable man to impart light into the HEARTS of others. The golden oil of love will flow freely, to shine out in good works, in real heartfelt service for GOD.

Because of Adam's sin in the garden every human since has been born into sin and therefore sin is a principal seated in the center and defiles the whole circuit of our actions. There is something on the inside of man of his own creating which can either tranquilize or traumatize him. It is a good or bad sense of right and wrong. Conscience, even though it sometimes torments, is very necessary; for without it man would be devoid of that capability which brings his premium joy, his own endorsement. Without conscience, man would not be man.

We can never repay the debt owed to the MASTER thus we should mark the sacredness of GOD'S gift by giving a portion of all we have to be set aside and dedicated to THE SUPREME BEING. When we fail this requirement of obedience our HEARTS will begin a hardening process, in refusing to obey to return just a little of what we have been given we move away from GOD'S intended purpose for our lives and into death. Our HEART grows more rigid, more sickly with each refusal to obey GOD'S Will. Our bodies become apathetic and our arteries a little more callous with each step away from GOD. Eventually our conscious mind will be overcome by the evil one [our enemy, GOD'S enemy] and we will not be able to function on a basis of ability to discern [tell or recognize] good from evil.

The enemy, this prince of darkness will have entered and seared [hardened,burned,destroyed] our mind to a point we no longer recognize the heavy chains of bondage that satan has wrapped us in and we will walk somewhat arrogant but none the less in fright, hatred, hostility, egotism and haughtiness, etc. We have been deceived and are held by the umbilical cord of our sin. When the enemy captures our life we need to bear in mind the reasons he comes, to steal, kill and destroy. This enemy will attack the weakened region first and slowly annihilate to the point of doom, he will control the organ of speech and prescribe suffering, shattering, damaging, confusion for all who love us or know us.

JAMES 3:8-11 THE TONGUE IS AN UNRULY EVIL FULL OF DEADLY POISON ETC. PROVERBS 12:18 THE TONGUE CAN BE LIKE A PIERCING SWORD. IT CAN CAUSE OUR FAILING AND OUR SICKNESS, BUT THE TONGUE OF THE WISE BRINGETH HEALTH.

Each time we speak we are building up or tearing down, blessing or cursing. There by introducing what we articulate as a prescription upon our selves in the form of condemnation that will bring about sickness, disease and discouragement.

MATTHEW 15:18-20 "WHAT COMES OUT OF YOUR MOUTH IS ACTUALLY COMING FROM YOUR HEART, AND THAT IS WHAT MAKES A PERSON UN-CLEAN. 19 FOR OUT OF THE HEART COME FORTH WICKED THOUGHTS, MURDER, ADULTERY AND OTHER KINDS OF SEXUAL IMMORALITY, THEFT, LIES, SLANDERS...20. THESE ARE WHAT REALLY MAKE A PERSON UNCLEAN, BUT EATING WITHOUT DOING RITUAL HAND WASHING DOES NOT MAKE A PERSON UNCLEAN."

Since it is impossible for us to separate the spirit from the flesh and that which effects the flesh also affects and reflects the spirit/soul, and vice-versa. GOD'S WORD like a dissecting knife will penetrate into our intermost being and will force a radical division and distinction between those who follow THE BIBLE and unbelievers. Our thoughts [mind] and HEART felt ideas [desires] will be brought under judgment and we will either follow THE LORD or seek death..

HIS WORD is nourishment to the soul in the same way that food is essential to the body and when we neglect to consume HIS WORD, we become spiritually weak and vulnerable to the monarch of hell and his evil spirits who move about with one intent in mind and that is to enter into the things of GOD to condemn the soul of GOD'S created Image. There by grieving our LORD YESHUA the MESSIAH, WHO died to save us.

Evil spirits cause unbelief and will bring on a spirit of discouragement in times of pressure and opposition. Our lack of confidence in GOD becomes disturbed and restless as a raging sea when our faith begins to fail, and our trust in GOD diminishes. We develop a disposition to complain and worry in the mist of pain and poverty and are overwhelmed by our feelings as doubt comes in. We can only please GOD by faith and we can only know faith by hearing.

So why do we choose to wonder out of HIS WORD? We are not the master of our own purpose, Humble heaven taught that believers have HIS Authority and will exercise free agency in GOD'S Spirit of dependence.

Seven {7} days without prayer makes one weak. After a short while of rejecting GOD, HIS WORD and conversation with HIM, our faith will become a 'religion', a formality of deadness. We will develop a lack of concern for the Will of GOD, a spirit of rebellion, pride, selfishness, and revenge will come forth to bankrupt this gift GOD gave us in our 'temple'. We won't be concerned if others know GOD and will become unable to understand how GOD'S Power, through HIS precious SON at Calvary has already defeated satan for our advantage. As we cherish the flesh we will justify our actions and revenge will be our utmost right. We will open wounds that will take vengeance and will cause disease and rot in our systems that will condemn our character.

Our divine health and protection can only be ministered when we remain faithful to GOD in the valley as well as on the hill top. Only GOD'S HOLY SPIRIT will enable us, by confession and faith to bring our 'selfishness' to the cross and put to death the carnal man. HIS HOLY SPIRIT will raise up the new man and to bestow upon us the new-fashioned HEART, free from the devils traits such as hardness, disease, jealousy, greed, worry, envy and the like.

It is urgent that we seek GOD so that we do not attempt to work out problems in the flesh, for without GOD we can not be wise in our dealings. Far to often we speak "the WORD" to others thinking we will make them change but our inner attitude is one of pride in the fact that 'we know the WORD' and thus the HOLY SPIRIT is thwarted. The fleshly spirit of those to whom we have so pridefully spoken senses that pride in us and GOD'S WILL is made of none effect. As HIS servant we need always to allow GOD to prepare the HEART of those to whom we plan to speak. Being sensitive to HIS gentle nudging before we verbalize will help us hear HIS Still Small Voice. HE may have another more effective message through our service, rather than through our mouth.

BUT WHY DOST THOU JUDGE THY BROTHER? OR WHY DOST THOU SET AT NAUGHT THY BROTHER? FOR WE SHALL ALL STAND BEFORE THE JUDGMENT SEAT OF CHRIST? ROMANS 14:4

Through the WORD only is man confronted by GOD where nothing can be concealed. We stand stripped, bear and fully exposed by HIS searching glance, as we come face to face with the Redeemer or judge, according to what we choose. When we abide in, read and inhale HIS living WORD [our spirit food] our faith becomes mounted upon the Rock of Salvation. Like the Eagle we begin to soar over our problem, seeing them through GOD'S eyes. No matter whether our enigma is health, finances, or any other thing, as we continue in HIS WORD our wisdom increases as does our strength and knowledge.

We will fully appreciate the responsibility we are under when we hear HIS WORD for it shares GOD'S attributes of GOD

HIMSELF. HE is always active in HIS WORD so it is never without result.

ISAIAH 55:11   SO SHALL MY WORD BE THAT GOETH FORTH OUT OF MY MOUTH; IT SHALL NOT RETURN UNTO ME VOID, BUT IT SHALL ACCOMPLISH THAT WHICH I PLEASE, AND IT SHALL PROSPER IN THE THING WHERETO I SENT IT.

As we stand in faith with GOD'S DIVINE protection we learn to overcome spiritual battles and with each new victory we become more dependent upon GOD. After a few victories we realize GOD'S DIVINE presence is our protection and to keep that ever present guardianship we must dwell upon the Rock by indulging in HIS WORD, proclaiming "IT" and making it our objective.

It is when we turn from GOD to seek our own frivolous gratification that we walk downward from HIS divine mount of safekeeping to fan idol worship. We move on to uncover the entrance of our HEART for the devil to penetrate. With each step away from GOD we tread further into satan's domain of idolatry and isms. [anarchy, vain imagination, satanism, communism, occultism, Buddhism, etc]. The worlds system harbors failure and horror as the HEARTS of men terminate themselves for fear.

LUKE 21:26 MEN'S HEARTS FAILING THEM FOR FEAR, AND FOR LOOKING AFTER THOSE THINGS WHICH ARE COMING ON THE EARTH; FOR THE POWERS OF HEAVEN SHALL BE SHAKEN

Only HIS WORD is alive and full of life and has power to achieve, It brings either salvation or judgment, depending on the condition of our HEART.. Our choice will cause either wellness or disease to begin.

When we hear GOD'S WORD with our whole HEART and are quick to cleave to "IT" in obedience, we will delight in the blessings HE guarantees in "IT". Only when we make a conscience decision to seek HIM in HIS WORD do we become vitally united to "IT" by means of faith. We will exhibit zeal and earnest endeavor in continual pursuit of GOD'S Will and thus have the OPPORTUNITY TO HEAR HIS VOICE. By our CHOICE WE BECOME SAVED OR LOST.

MATTHEW 7:24-27 "SO EVERYONE WHO HEARS THESE WORDS OF MINE AND ACTS ON THEM WILL BE LIKE A SENSIBLE MAN WHO BUILT HIS HOUSE ON BEDROCK. THE RAIN FELL, THE RIVERS FLOODED, THE WINDS BLEW AND BEAT AGAINST THAT HOUSE, BUT IT DIDN'T COLLAPSE, BECAUSE ITS FOUNDATION WAS ON ROCK. 26. BUT EVERYONE WHO HEARS THESE WORDS OF MINE AND DOES NOT ACT ON THEM WILL BE LIKE A STUPID MAN WHO BUILT HIS HOUSE ON SAND. 27. THE RAIN FELL. THE RIVERS FLOODED, THE WIND BLEW AND BEAT AGAINST THAT HOUSE, AND IT COLLAPSED, AND ITS COLLAPSE WAS HORRENDOUS!" JEWISH NEW TESTAMENT}

Disobedience is unbelief and doubt is death. Thus the un-believer is spiritually dead, "DEAD IN TRESPASSES AND SINS". Faith from the un-believer is not possible because a dead man can not believe anything. Therefore it is impossible for them who are in the flesh to please GOD. It is an invigorating experience to hear someone speak of the positive power of their faith for they come not seeking answers, but praising GOD for his wisdom and solutions. They were loyal to pursue GOD'S Way instead of mans and because of their submission to GOD'S WORD they received a divine manifestation. Their face beams with confidence and joy and refreshes all who are witness. The simple truth is that they sought to find answers from GOD through HIS WORD, not the world.

ROMANS 8:8 THUS, THOSE WHO IDENTIFY WITH THEIR OLD NATURE CAN NOT PLEASE GOD."

The work of GOD'S HOLY SPIRIT is 'quickening' to one who is dead in sin. It always precedes faith in CHRIST the MESSIAH just as cause precedes effect. When the heart turns to THE MESSIAH[CHRIST] by the SPIRIT the SAVIOUR is immediately embraced by the sinner. Thus the mind becomes free of trouble & doubts and will be saved from unbelief.

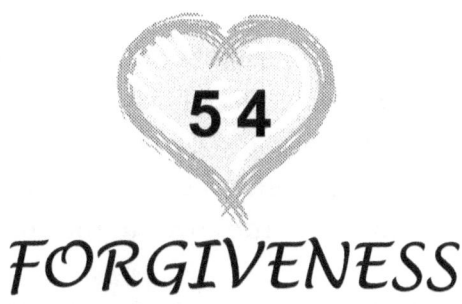

FORGIVENESS

Forgiveness has two directions in our life. From HIS forgiveness to us we must extend forgiveness to others. It is a condition of our forgiveness that we must be able and capable and willing to forgive others as HE has forgiven us. Great psychological implications of sin are removed when we practice forgiveness of others.

Guilt is a major cause of stress and our conscious mind is often couched in unfor-giveness. Our knowing right from wrong always condemns our wrong, even when others are unaware of our wrong doing. Unforgiveness = guilt = stress = pain = friction = disease. If our initial impulse is to hide guilt by silence, that secrecy over comes our wisdom to confess or forgive. It is thrust in to our subconscious to seep out in symptoms of mental and physical distress, an effective tool of satan. We are chained [invisible] into a major crisis of brain or HEART problems, arthritis, cancer, etc. Groaning and complaining becomes a character of our daily menu. We develop deep seated pain and involuntary groans of the bodies as our problems become a mass of disharmony while the conscience continuanually pleads to confess and be clean, is blindly or willingly ignored. Our obstinate persistence in the repression of our sub-conscious has reduced our vigor like the withering of a tree in a prolonged drought.

For our healing, the turning point will come when we humbly confess to GOD our sin, rebellion, disobedience [transgressions], and our inward corruption [iniquity]. When and if we allow GOD to come in to cleanse and renew our HEART, cover our sin, then the enemy will move out of our temple to stop the torment of guilt, stress,anguish, pain, disease. We allowed our sin to become an issue between us and our GOD when we move away from HIM who is our GOD by attempting to cover our shame, guilt, and sin with fig leaves. When in reality the more we wrap ourselves in rebellion, the more room we turn over to the enemy for our own destruction.

Distress will affect our soul and body. Our HEART feels and records everything and our misery will give rise to anxiety and uncertainty. We become suspicious and our life is withered by misgivings of even our acquaintances, it will shake even the loyalty of our closest friend.

Another avenue of forgiveness is our own, toward our brother who has wronged us. It begins with hurt feelings of having been wronged or not agreed with. Our pride rises up with a 'who do they think they are' attitude, as if we are the ultimate authority in that situation. We never stop to consider 'they' may have had a different experience and see the same situation from a opposite viewpoint. In essence we will not be forgiven unless we choose to forgive others. By repentance we enter a new sphere of divine protection amid the storms of life.

LUKE 13:3 NO I TELL YOU. RATHER, UNLESS YOU TURN TO GOD FROM YOUR SINS, YOU WILL ALL DIE AS THEY DID. :4 OR WHAT ABOUT THOSE EIGHTEEN PEOPLE WHO DIED WHEN THE TOWER AT SHILOACH FELL ON THEM? DO YOU THINK THEY WERE WORSE OFFENDERS THAN

ALL THE OTHER PEOPLE LIVING IN YERUSHALAYIM? {JERUSALEM} :5 NO, I TELL YOU. RATHER UNLESS YOU TURN FROM YOUR SINS, YOU WILL ALL DIE SIMILARLY. JEWISH NEW TESTAMENT

Upon repentance and forgiveness of others our guilt is replaced by the divine WORD of sympathetic guidance. YESHUA - The divine counselor steps in and replaces our self righteousness with GOD Righteousness and healing is completed, instantly the bond between Father and child is restored. If we refuse forgiveness, we choose pride and arrogance and our HEART becomes defiant, unteachable and stubborn. If we refuse to draw near to GOD in sweet submission, the FATHER will discipline us by judgment.

It is the sin that we allow that causes us to turn from GOD, and uncontrollable sin brings judgment or compassion. Our selection lies in our decision to confess and be cleansed in pure delight that springs from a guileless HEART, in which peace is inseparable from purity or to vindicate ourselves and go on the defensive, disputing GOD'S Will in which case HE will ultimately bring judgment upon us.

As pride grows, we move away from GOD thereby allowing entry to satan whose demons flood in to feed our frenzied conceit. This monarch from hell and his demons endeavor to make sure we are on the correct course of attack by turning our haughtiness to anger even exalting our position from brother to judge.

2 THESE. 2:13 "BUT WE HAVE TO KEEP THANKING GOD FOR YOU ALWAYS, BROTHERS WHOM THE LORD LOVES, BECAUSE GOD CHOSE YOU AS FIRST FRUITS FOR DELIVERANCE BY GIVING YOU THE HOLINESS THAT HAS ITS ORIGIN IN THE SPIRIT AND THE FAITHFULNESS THAT HAS ITS ORIGIN IN THE TRUTH." JEWISH NEW TESTAMENT

"Entrance of THY WORD giveth Light" The BIBLE is a lamp and a light. There is only one road to eternal life and the Bible guides us through the rough places, steep hills, thorns, briars, and across deep waters. As we begin our journey we must submit totally to YESHUA and allow HIS Holy Spirit to quietly teach, lead and guide us. Patience, study, and obedience, must be our main stay for they will gently escort us in peace to nothing doubting in GOD.

55

THE REFINING FIRE

PROVERBS 17:3 "THE FINING POT IS FOR SILVER AND THE FURNACE FOR GOLD, BUT THE LORD TRIETH THE HEARTS."

GOD treasures each of HIS creations of mankind who are made in HIS Image and HE places our value above that of gold. HE likens each of us to a superlative gold piece fit for purification so that we may assume HIS WILL to be fitted for HIS KINGDOM in Eternity. Just as iniquity captivates the sinner before repentance that delivers one to the furnace, dross cleaves inseparably to gold but the refiner's process burns and purifies and only the most precious of gold is all that is left for use. All the useless dross is burned away. Consequently just as gold is put into a furnace to separate the dross from the pure and precious metal, so too is the carnal Christian or the un-believer allowed to go through the furnace in test of faith to separate the good from the evil. Faith like gold is invisible to the workman's eye before placed into the furnace. After the purging of the heat and separation from the sin [dross]we become beautifully redeemed. It is only after we submit our lives to HIM and go through the purification process, that we are made fit for use in the MASTER'S SERVICE.

The refining process is slow but the results are sure and nothing but evil dross will perish. The vilest lump can be turned into the finest gold, so, to the HEART under the all knowing eyes of GOD.

"HIS EYES WERE AS A FLAME OF FIRE."   REV. 1:14b

Nothing deceives HIM nor escapes HIS probing search. HE searches for the willing HEART of obedience. Submission to GOD'S Will is the secret of success in our health, business, marriage, family, recreation, in all areas of nature. The tormented man must always examine his conscience for offense that provokes GOD, and he must petition for benevolence and restoration. Human torment and hostility are the outward expressions of divine disapproval and will elevate stress that is an un-natural friction of the system, that will eventually cause pain and in due time disease.

JERE 9:7, "THEREFORE THUS SAITH THE LORD OF HOSTS, BEHOLD I WILL MELT THEM AND TRY THEM; FOR HOW SHALL I DO FOR THE DAUGHTER OF MY PEOPLE?   9:8 THEIR TONGUE IS AN ARROW SHOT OUT; IT SPEAKETH DECEIT; ONE SPEAKETH PEACEABLY TO HIS NEIGHBOR WITH HIS MOUTH, BUT IN HEART HE LAYETH HIS WAIT. 9:9   SHALL I NOT VISIT THEM FOR THESE THINGS ? SAITH THE LORD; SHALL NOT MY SOUL BE AVENGED ON SUCH.

None of us know ourselves until GOD reveals HIS Law to our HEART. A process of obedience, as one step is placed upon another that is pleasing to our LORD. Wisdom is a learning procedure that is accessible only to those who select to behave according to GOD'S Will.

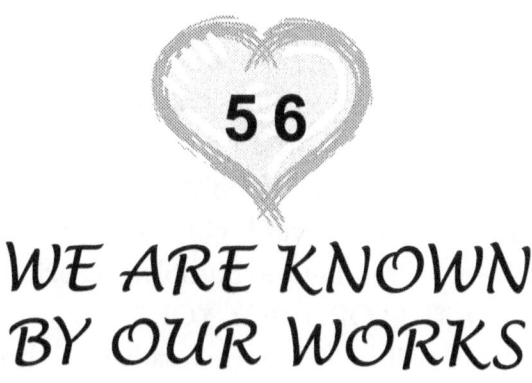

WE ARE KNOWN
BY OUR WORKS

1 COR. 3:13 "EVERY MAN'S WORK SHALL BE MADE MANIFEST; FOR THE DAY SHALL DECLARE IT, BECAUSE IT SHALL BE REVEALED BY FIRE; AND THE FIRE SHALL TRY EVERY MAN'S WORK OF WHAT SORT IT IS."

Only GOD can purge our HEART and make it free from sin, any endeavor we compose is futile for no man has ever had the omnipotence to transpose himself. Only GOD'S refining eyes and HIS redeeming unchanging Will can:

[1] cause hidden evil to be exposed for humiliation,

[2] cause hidden good be exposed to honor,

[3] reflect the plague of our own heart.

Only through GOD can we perceive the concealed transgressions that are secluded in the indentation of our HEARTS, our subconscious is sprinkled over with time and lost memories of past hurts and pains, pigeonholed and hopefully forgotten.

Only GOD fathoms & comprehends the every day slings and arrows that explode in our HEART. The immense distinction is in the manner we yield to them and allow the unpredictable changes to effect us. We can opt to let go by permitting GOD to manage them or we can proceed in "our own wisdom" to plunge into them. GOD assigns tribulations for examination of our HEART for the purpose of rooting out, revealing, and diminishing the secret evil concealed within each of us.

HIS WORD is a piercing furnace that will personify to us our accountability and unworthiness of HIS majestic notice. We will come to realize the unmerited favor we have with HIM and wonder why HE would send HIS only SON to die for such as we are. HIS purging is a painful yet highly necessary process of fire which makes the flesh tremble and humbles the prideful, unwilling HEART to say "NOT I LORD, BUT YOU".

The distinction will be made as we advance through the fire and how we change in response to the LORD. Will we go through the furnace as the three Hebrew boys, with our eyes firmly fixed upon YESHUA? Will we come through without even the faint smell of fire, blessed and glorified by GOD, or will we come out in anger and bitterness, mad at GOD for allowing us to be subjected to such a fire? Shall we not commit as gold without dross, in well grounded confidence to HIS Wisdom, tenderness & love?

JERE 10:24 OH LORD, CORRECT ME, WITH JUDGMENT, NOT IN THINE ANGER, LEST THOU BRING ME TO NOTHING.

Only the best of material for praise is brought to light out of a consecrated furnace. We must cautiously investigate, lest we perceive the value of these trying dispensations in disbelief thereby causing our pain and discomfort to attack our spirit and drive away the HOLY SPIRIT by our fleshly justification. We must remember that torment and burdens are glitches in our spirit to be checked and guarded against through HIS WORD the DIVINE

PLAN. If left unchecked it will create disease by friction which is unnatural to we who are made in HIS Image.

As the gold is purged from metal to be come perfect, we are also purged by our trails. GODLY results will melt away our stubborn will and remove our worldly idols of self interest and we will seek HIM with the entireness of our HEART. Just as gold comes from the furnace so shall we come as a useful, radiant and brighter gem. In time, we will come out of great afflictions to become more glorious with grace and splendor. We will become sterling in quality if GOD is allowed to do the purging of our HEART.

As we proceed through the furnace GOD will not let us slip away if our HEART is turned toward HIM. Even when we blunder and make mistakes - HE sits, watching and gently wooing our HEART back to HIM. It is when we resist, demand, and justify, our ungodly way that our HEART becomes hardened and little by little as we journey down the road of 'self' the HEART moves away from GOD'S DIVINE PLAN for our lives. As we slowly move away our HEART becomes a little harder with each denial.

Suddenly we realize, our HEART is so hardened it has turned like stone and there is no way blood can channel through it. It is suited with disease and we are geared for a 'HEART ATTACK'! We repose in wonderment of what has happened? Why is GOD allowing this to befall us, when in essence, He has allowed nothing to happen. It was we who migrated beyond HIS Perfect Will away from HIS Divine Covering; the concealment that GOD, HIMSELF sacrificed HIS only SON to die for.

We have make sport of the great payment GOD made for our Salvation, shook our clenched hand into HIS FACE with our "egotistical disposition", and anticipated that HE would give rise to particular preparations for us? When it was our iniquity that provoked our stiffness of HEART, our HEART plague, and our HEART attack.

MALACHI 3:2-3   BUT WHO MAY ABIDE THE DAY OF HIS COMING? AND WHO SHALL STAND WHEN HE APPEARETH? FOR HE IS LIKE A REFINER'S FIRE & LIKE FULLER'S SOAP;   :3 AND HE SHALL SIT AS A REFINER AND PURIFIER OF SILVER; :4 AND HE SHALL PURIFY THE SONS OF LEVI AND PURGE THEM AS GOLD AND SILVER, THAT THEY MAY OFFER THE LORD AN OFFERING IN RIGHTEOUSNESS.

If we embrace YESHUA, righteousness will come from our HEART. It will be found on our lips and known by our actions as well as our countenance. It will be composed on the walls of our dwelling, our business and even on our gate post. As we surrender to HIS WILL, HE observes patiently ,ceaselessly and ready to protect us. For GOD is the source of right {Deut. 1:17}, judge of all the earth. It is inconceivable that HE should not do right {Gen. 18:25} or that HE would pervert justice {Job 8:3} or that HE could do wickedly {Job 34:12} FOR THE LORD IS A GOD OF JUSTICE {Isa 30:18} THE LORD IS RIGHTEOUS, HE LOVES RIGHTEOUSNESS {PS 11:7}

Righteousness goes beyond justice. Justice is strict and exact, giving each person his due. Righteousness implies benevolence, kindness, generosity.   Justice is form, a state of equilibrium; righteousness has a substantive associated meaning. Justice may be legal; righteousness is associated with a burning compassion for the oppressed. The theme of justice was not equal justice but a bias in favor of the poor and it was to also lean toward mercy for the widows and orphans. However justice dies when dehumanized, no matter how exactly it may be exercised it dies when consecrated for beyond all justice is GOD'S compassion. The logic of justice may seem impersonal but the concern for it is an act of love.

ZACH. 13:9 AND I WILL BRING THE 3RD PART THROUGH THE FIRE AND WILL REFINE THEM AS SILVER IS REFINED,

AND WILL TRY THEM AS GOLD IS TRIED; THEY SHALL CARRY ON MY NAME AND I WILL HEAR THEM; I WILL SAY, IT IS MY PEOPLE AND THEY SHALL SAY, THE LORD IS MY GOD.

Every second of our trial is above gold and is always allowed to purify our HEART for a richer vein in GOD'S attainment. We then learn to appreciate our suffering SAVIOUR as HE becomes more realized and endeared. We will become grounded and established in our confidence of our ONE and only true GOD. In the furnace we will see the seal of our election if we endure.

ISAIAH 48:10 BEHOLD, I HAVE REFINED THEE, BUT NOT WITH SILVER; I HAVE CHOSEN THEE IN THE FURNACE OF AFFLICTION.

Our anticipation of our LORD, appearing as we dwell in the furnace, will be made into a crown of pure gold and be found unto praise, honour and glory. We express trust in GOD'S order by being ever thankful, thus obedience becomes a sideline of that trust, even when we feel that thanking GOD is absolutely opposed to our will and seems ridiculous. It's often a test of faith and HIS Will is above all we can know or understand.

2 THESS. 5:18 GIVE THANKS IN ALL CIRCUMSTANCES, FOR THIS IS GOD'S WILL FOR "US" YOU IN YESHUA.

END